THE HEALING PATH OF PRAYER

THE HEALING PATH OF PRAYER

A MODERN MYSTIC'S GUIDE TO SPIRITUAL POWER

RON ROTH

WITH PETER OCCHIOGROSSO

FOREWORD BY CAROLINE MYSS, Ph.D.

THREE RIVERS PRESS/NEW YORK

Grateful acknowledgment is made to the following for permission to reprint: Bear & Co., Santa Fe, New Mexico, for excerpts from *Illuminations of Hildegard of Bingen*, with commentary by Matthew Fox, copyright © 1985; Donadio and Ashworth, Inc., and Harcourt Brace & Company for excerpts from *Sister Aimee* by Daniel Mark Epstein, copyright © 1993 by Daniel Mark Epstein; Element Books, Inc., for excerpts from *The New Living Qabalah* by Will Parfitt, copyright © 1988, 1995 by Will Parfitt; HarperCollins Publishers, Inc., for excerpts from *Desert Wisdom: Middle Eastern Sacred Writing* by Neil Douglas-Klotz, copyright © 1995 by Neil Douglas-Klotz; HarperCollins Publishers, Inc., for excerpts from #67 from *Tao te Ching* translated by Stephen Mitchell, translation copyright © 1988 by Stephen Mitchell; The Lockman Foundation for scripture taken from the *Amplified® New Testament*, copyright © 1954, 1958, 1987 by The Lockman Foundation; Paragon House, St. Paul, Minnesota, for excerpts from *World Scriptures: A Comparative Anthology of Sacred Texts* edited by Andrew Wilson, copyright © 1995 by Paragon House; Self-Realization Fellowship, Los Angeles, California, for excerpts from *Man's Eternal Quest* by Paramahansa Yogananda, copyright © 1982; Simon & Schuster and Elizabeth K. Stratton, M.S., for excerpts from *Touching Spirit: A Journey of Healing and Personal Resurrection* by Elizabeth K. Stratton, M.S., copyright © 1996 by Elizabeth K. Stratton, M.S.

Published by Three Rivers Press, a division of Crown Publishers, Inc., 201 East 50th Street, New York, New York 10022

Originally published in hardcover by Harmony Books, a division of Crown Publishers, Inc., in 1997

Random House, Inc. New York, Toronto, London, Sydney, Auckland
www.randomhouse.com

Three Rivers Press and colophon are trademarks of Crown Publishers, Inc.

Printed in the United States of America

Design by June Bennett-Tantillo

Library of Congress Cataloging-in-Publication Data
Roth, Ron.
The healing path of prayer : a modern mystic's guide to spiritual power / by Ron Roth with Peter Occhiogrosso ; foreword by Caroline Myss.—1st ed.
Includes bibliographical references and index.
1. Spiritual healing. 2. Healing—Religious aspects.
3. Mysticism. 4. Prayer. 5. Spiritual exercises.
I. Occhiogrosso, Peter. II. Title.
BL65.M4R68   1997
291.4'3—dc21   97-16801

ISBN 0-609-80226-7

10 9 8 7 6 5 4 3 2 1

First Paperback Edition

*To all the friends and family members who supported me as
I traveled my own path of prayer, from institutional to independent
healer. Your love helped bring me closer to God during a time
of difficulty and growth.*

ACKNOWLEDGMENTS

I am indebted to many people whose love, support, and encouragement during my years of healing work have brought me to this joyous moment in my life, culminating in the realization of this book. Although they are too numerous to list, I am grateful to each of them, and I ask God to bless them all with the best life has to offer. I do, however, need to single out a handful of people who were instrumental in helping me complete this book.

I begin by thanking my Aunt Julie and Uncle Ben and my associate and dearest friend, Paul Funfsinn, whose guidance and love continue to be invaluable assets to me. Caroline Myss was there for me during my darkest times of loneliness. Dr. Norman Shealy encouraged me to move forward in the field of spiritual healing. Bob and Linda Sendra have given me their friendship and inspiration throughout the years. My parents, William and Valerie, have passed from the physical dimension of existence, yet their spirit is continually with me.

Louise L. Green was my first office manager and secretary in healing work, and her combination of guidance and efficiency kept my healing ministry on its course during the early days. Dorothy and Karl Baughman opened their home to me and my work so that I could continue to bring God's healing love to an even larger number of people. Janice Christopher and Eugenia Patthoff assisted me in assembling the original manuscript.

I would also like to thank my agent, Stuart Krichevsky, who shepherded this project through the publishing stage, and my editor, Leslie Meredith, who had faith in this book from the beginning and whose many helpful suggestions improved the manuscript immensely. Finally, I want to thank my coauthor, Peter Occhiogrosso, whose expertise in Eastern religions and mysticism have brought me to a deeper appreciation of these traditions. He has become more than a colleague to me. I call him my friend.

CONTENTS

CONTENTS

FOREWORD
Caroline Myss, Ph.D.

Does prayer really work or are we simply releasing our needs and concerns into empty space? How do we know our prayers are answered? Are miracles real? If so, do we need to do something special to qualify for such profound divine intervention?

Few of us have not asked these types of questions. Everyone of us has had moments—perhaps even years—when we have been unable to find a way through the crises that are a continual part of the human experience. After all, life is a mystery and we all require a candle to light our way through the dark times.

The Healing Path of Prayer: A Modern Mystic's Guide to Spiritual Power is a treasury of answers to these questions—answers that we can rarely attain on our own. Those who have received responses to their prayers say with absolute certainty that the source of their answer was divine and believe that all is possible with faith. How do we find our faith? Is there a way to activate this force inside of us when we need it?

In this rich and inspiring book, Ron guides us into the heart of prayer and offers us examples of profound healings that can result from prayer—from the healing of terminal illnesses to the healing of infertility. These remarkable real-life events are all a part of Ron's life as a healer and of all that he represents as a teacher of the mysteries of God.

In reading this magnificent book, you know immediately that each story Ron shares is authentic, separating the meaning and power of prayer from the fictitious and superstitious notions that often clutter the truth. He directs us into the power of these experiences by weaving personal instructions on how to pray using meditation techniques with directions on how to use our breath to draw us into the interior of our minds, our hearts, and our spirits. The techniques in this book are both ancient and modern, universal and personal. Moreover, they are effective. Aside from the many methods of instruction Ron presents, he also shares with us the history of prayer, such as the original wording and meaning of the "Our Father," offering us insight into how we were meant to interpret that prayer. Knowing the truth behind this prayer and the many others he investigates can literally bring you to your knees with the awesome light he shines on the history of these sacred words and the power they contain—power that was and is meant to flood our spiritual life.

Ron further adds so much wealth to his work by combining the teachings of other major spiritual traditions. His use of the endless wisdom of the Hebrew tradition, together with that of Hinduism and Buddhism, complete his presentation like a mandala, giving us a spectrum of light and truth through which to absorb the intimate and ever-compassionate nature of God.

I feel honored to be a part of this text with this Foreword, not only because Ron is one of my dearest friends, but because I have personally witnessed the power of prayer he describes, as well as his God-given ability to heal others. Throughout this affecting and effective teaching, Ron shares his personal journey as a Catholic priest who discovered the reality of divine intervention in healing. Although Ron had never planned a life as a healer, he was called to the task in the manner that God often calls us—when we least expect it and in such a way that we cannot say no. He was called on spontaneously and publicly to pray, and when he did members of the prayer service were healed. Were someone to ask me if Ron's healing power is authentic, I would have no other reply but yes. And if someone asked me to describe in one word the significance of this book, only one word is worthy of reply: truth.

AUTHOR'S NOTE

My whole mission is to make the idea of a loving God credible again to people. For too long, religion has portrayed a punishing God, lying in wait to throw the wicked into hell for breaking even one of His laws. I want to spread the word that God is on our side.

The basis of this book is the knowledge that every one of us has at one time or another felt an energy that we didn't know how to explain. In our most ecstatic moments, we may have felt a touch on our shoulder, and nobody was there. We may have felt some caring presence breathing upon us, and no one was there. We may have smelled the aroma of roses when none were in the room. In my case, when I went to Medjugorje the chain of the rosary I was praying on turned to gold. These phenomena are evidence of God's love in action, saying to us that there is energy all around us that we haven't yet tapped into. When we finally do learn to tap into that energy through prayer, it will work wonders. . . .

INTRODUCTION

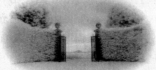

*Don't you know that you yourselves are God's temple
and that God's Spirit lives in you?*

◆

1 Corinthians 3:16

According to the Gospel of John, Jesus said to his disciples (14:12), "Truly, truly, I say to you, he who believes in me will also do the works that I do; and greater works than these will he do." What did Jesus actually mean by these startling words? Was he saying that we would share an abstract piety, or did he mean that we could all possess the ability to heal, as he did? I believe that Jesus meant exactly what he said when he told his disciples, "Whoever says to this mountain, 'Be taken up and cast into the sea,' and does not doubt in his heart, but believes that what he says will come to pass, it will be done for him" (Mark 11:23–24).

Jesus is referring to the faith that results in healing. Clearly he is not referring to faith in institutional dogmas and doctrines—in fact, Jesus spent much of his ministry decrying the institutional brand of faith purveyed by the religious leaders of his day. Repeatedly in the Gospels, Jesus names personal, inner faith as the immediate cause of the miraculous. "Daughter, your faith has made you well," he says to the woman who touched the hem of his garment and was healed of her hemorrhaging (Mark 5:24ff). "Go your way; your faith has made you whole," he says to the blind beggar (Luke 18:42). When the Roman centurion's servant is miraculously healed, Jesus does not tell the centurion that God has healed his servant, or even that he (Jesus) has healed him. The centurion's faith, Jesus says, has saved his servant.

In the verse following his statement about moving mountains in Mark 11, Jesus tells us plainly: "Whatever you ask in prayer, you will receive if you have faith." As elsewhere in the Gospels, Jesus links prayer with the ability to heal and produce miracles. But he adds one crucial condition: "Whenever you stand praying, forgive, if you have anything against anyone; so that your Father also who is in heaven will forgive you your trespasses." Jesus' mission is to transmit love and forgiveness, which are prerequisites to authentic prayer.

Faith, prayer, forgiveness. These are the linchpins of the teachings of Jesus of Nazareth. If we but knew how to pray and had faith that what we were praying for would come to be, Jesus is telling us, we could ourselves perform the same feats as he—and more. We can heal ourselves and others, we can bring abundance and joy to our lives—but first we have to learn how to pray. In this book, I will attempt to explain in detail the connection between healing, faith, and prayer, and give explicit instructions on how you can pray in a way that taps into the healing energy of God. That energy can be applied not only toward physical healing but also, perhaps more significantly, to heal emotional and spiritual wounds that have thrown the spirit out of balance and may have opened the door for physical maladies. On a larger scale, we can look at our entire life as one long healing process: as we heal ourselves of our identification with the body and the separative ego, we learn to see ourselves as spirit connected with all other human spirits and with the Spirit of God. This is indeed healing toward wholeness.

In some cases, simply reconceptualizing how you perceive God and how you approach prayer may release you from the negative energy generated by the confused and often oppressive conceptions that may have been inculcated in you by religious institutions earlier in life. Such a reconception in itself may begin the healing of body, mind, and spirit.

Through a series of simple but effective daily practices and rituals, you can become your own priest and celebrate your own sacraments. You can become a mystic in the course of your daily life. Today you no longer need to enter a convent or seminary, a monastery or ashram or temple, to live the mystical life. By learning how to pray effectively and how to gain access to the healing energy of God, we can all be mystics and priests. We will be fulfilling the promise in the ancient scripture of Exodus, which predates the teachings of Jesus, and which says, in the nineteenth chapter, that God led his people out of Egypt and bore them "on eagles' wings" to make them His own if they keep His covenant. Then God adds, "For all the earth is mine, and you shall be to me a kingdom of priests and a holy nation."

I believe it is our calling today to be a kingdom of priests. Without the mediation of an institutional church, we can all take on the functions of priest and laity, and practice faith, prayer, and forgiveness. In fact, that artificial division between official and layperson is no longer necessary. I'd like to propose a single category for all of us: mystic.

To that end, I've included in each chapter of this book distinctive prayer and meditation exercises that each of you can incorporate into your lives. Some take more time than others; some should be performed alone, while others can be conducted with a friend or a group of like-minded souls. But all are designed to be worked into your daily schedule so that you can maximize your awareness and remembrance of the divine presence in your life. Although I invite you to find your own rhythm in working with these exercises, I would recommend that you allow at least a week for each of them to enter gently into your consciousness. It's easy to become confused or feel overwhelmed by taking on too much spiritual work too quickly. If you read the book at a faster pace than that, give yourself time to return to the exercises you've passed over once you've incorporated the previous ones into your awareness. Naturally, you are free to stay with one particular prayer or exercise until you feel comfortable moving on, or at any time to take a rest from the process. It simply takes some people longer than others to digest each step along the path, depending on how long it takes your spirit to metabolize each prayer exercise. Nobody is keeping score.

People often express confusion over the difference between prayer and meditation. I've heard the saying that prayer is talking to God, but meditation is God talking to you. I don't agree with that, since for me prayer also means primarily listening to God. As far as I'm concerned, all prayer can be defined as communion with God in whatever form you choose, including silence. Meditation, then, is simply a particularized form of prayer.

If you have never meditated before, the best way to begin is by emptying your mind of any preconceptions you may have acquired, especially the notion that it takes years of hard work to "learn" how to meditate. You will actually begin to learn the moment you sit down and enter into one of the exercises in this book. All you really need is to find a quiet spot—preferably a separate room but possibly just a corner of your bedroom—and allot a few minutes each day during which you will not be disturbed.

Dozens of books on the market offer detailed instructions about posture and breathing—and someday I'm going to read them all, really I am. For now, it's best to keep the basics simple. Although it's helpful to sit up (lying down tends to be a prelude to sleep) and keep your back straight, you don't need to work yourself into a classic full-lotus posture. Especially for us aging Westerners with weak backs and crabby knees, sitting on a chair with your feet planted flat on the floor and legs uncrossed is fine. Closing your eyes is optional, and taking air in slowly and steadily through the nostrils and letting it out evenly through the mouth is the simplest and most common method.

Before doing anything else in your prayer or meditation sessions, spend a few minutes just placing your attention on your breath. Focusing on the breath is one element common to the meditation techniques of all the world's mystical traditions, whether Hindu, Buddhist, Taoist, Sufi, Kabbalistic, or Christian. As we shall see, the breath is one manifestation of the action of the Holy Spirit in the world. Some people like to place a few sacred images (we'll say more about those later), and possibly a candle or two on the floor or a low table that can serve as a home altar. One of the oldest forms of meditation from India involves focusing your attention on a candle flame, and this may help you in the beginning.

That's about all you need to know about meditation to get started. I'll provide somewhat more detailed advice beginning with the exercise at the end of Chapter 1.

It's natural for someone picking up a book of this kind, which purports to prescribe the most productive ways to pray, to wonder how I myself conceptualize the Divine. I'm afraid I can't answer that easily or succinctly, and I don't think it would be especially helpful even if I could. In the view of most Eastern mystics, we're wasting our time trying to define God; for them, God has to be experienced, and I would agree with them. My experience of God is of a loving Being of unbounded energy whose love and guidance are always available to me as long as I let myself be open to them.

My deepest aspiration for anyone reading this book is for each of you, through the exercises and prayers I've included, to find God in a way that is significant to you at this particular time in your life. I don't necessarily want you to have my experience of God, or your mother's or father's. You have to discover God on your own. That's part of what I believe Jesus was trying to get across when he said, "But when you pray, go into your closet and shut the door and pray to your Father who is in secret" (Matt. 6:6). You may gain great strength from praying or meditating with other people at times, but your experience of God will ultimately be your own. Think of it as a voyage of discovery, with the destination to become clearer as you sail further along.

IN THE
BEGINNING . . .

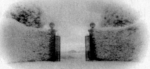

*My nature became so sensitized that I could lay my hands on any
man or woman and tell what organ was diseased, and to what extent.*

◆

JOHN LAKE

My first healing occurred when I was eleven years old. I had developed a severe strep throat and become so sick that my parents were getting ready to take me to the hospital. As I waited to go, I heard a voice inside me say very clearly, "Take your first two fingers and put them up to your throat where the infection is, and I will heal you."

I never doubted for a moment that this would happen. With a child's confidence, I did as I was told and immediately began to feel better. My parents told me not to speak of this to anyone, just as they had told me not to speak of an experience six years before, when, following a routine mastoid operation, something had gone wrong and I'd started turning blue. On that occasion, my throat had puffed up and the doctors had held out no hope that I would live. In referring to this incident later, my parents always told me that I had almost died of complications following surgery, but now I am convinced that I *had* died. I still retain a dim memory of seeing myself as a little child being taken into Jesus' arms and then abruptly pulled back to Earth. (When I was fifty-four, I recounted these events to a spiritually oriented psychiatrist friend of mine who told me that I had had a near-death experience. Until then, I simply hadn't had the vocabulary to describe it.)

When the healing occurred at age eleven, I didn't connect it to the earlier experience, and soon forgot both events until I was in my mid-thirties. By then, I had been a Roman Catholic priest for six years, having been ordained in 1966. Something had begun to happen in my work for which I wasn't prepared but that conjured up long-suppressed memories of those childhood events. The context couldn't have been more mundane, and perhaps the very ordinariness of the setting helped to set off in dramatic relief the surprising nature of what was about to occur. I had been assigned to outlying Midwestern parishes, safely ensconced among the corn and soybeans, where my superiors probably figured I couldn't disturb anyone with my somewhat iconoclastic views of the importance of individual spiritual authority. My work had begun to lose its savor, and I found myself increasingly ill at ease with my role as parish priest.

Around this time, a fellow priest named Dan with whom I had been in the seminary but who was a few years younger than I appeared in my parish. He had had a nervous breakdown some time before, yet when he visited me I saw that every pore of his being radiated a joy that I had lost. I had known him a long time and now he was utterly changed, so I asked him how he had come by this sudden joy.

"I had an experience with God," he said simply. When I asked how that had happened, he said that while he had been institutionalized some religious people had come to visit and had prayed with him. He said they had laid hands on him and asked God to give him just what he needed. And he got it. As a priest, of course, I ought to have believed in the power of prayer as much as anyone, but I had never seen such a simple and unavoidable sign of its efficacy. I asked Dan to pray with me as those folks had prayed with him. I still had enough faith to believe that something would come of it.

Dan told me to kneel down and then he uttered a prayer to God that completely astonished me. Dan's prayer may sound inexplicably simple, but all he said was "Come, Holy Spirit, fill Ron now." Then he began to speak in tongues—an unspecified language made up of uncomprehended and apparently random vocal sounds. The combination had a profound emotional and spiritual effect on me. I thought I knew how to pray. I thought I knew how to make a connection with God. I thought I understood that God was loving and merciful and kind, and was not a wrathful God. Yet when Dan spoke that prayer, something inexplicable happened to me. Today I would say that my heart chakra opened, because I could actually feel the heat and movement in my chest, and the one thing I wanted more than anything else at that moment was to give people an awareness of God's love. I had been pretty successful as a give-'em-hell preacher in the past, but all of that changed in a heart-beat. At the time, however, I did not know anything about the chakras, the seven spiritual energy centers in the body, derived from Hindu spirituality.

I felt this love within me so powerfully that I decided that I would try something different in my church. That Saturday, I called in the janitor at my church and asked him if he had a long microphone cord that could reach from the altar to the back of the church. He sounded dubious but he agreed to set it up for me. When I walked into the church on Sunday morning, for the first time in my preaching career I became aware of a presence taking hold of me. This presence took the form of an enveloping aura of confidence that told me to move away from the altar because I didn't need the notes I'd prepared for my sermon. If I would just allow myself to be a channel, what needed to be said to the people would be said.

If you've ever spent much time inside a Catholic church, you know that on a Sunday, most of the congregation arrives two minutes before mass and occupies the last ten pews in the back of the church. They fight for those rear pews, where they can hide without fear of being noticed. I felt that, if nothing else worked, just the fact that I could now walk to the back of the church where the parishioners didn't expect me to go would be enough to blow the saddle right out from underneath them. As I started to talk, sharing whatever was coming through me, I picked the microphone off its stand and made my way to the back. People who had been checking their wristwatches a moment before suddenly sat up straight with some alarm and began to listen. The following week, a small miracle occurred: most of my parishioners sat in the front. Maybe they felt that if I was going to the back of the church, they could avoid me by moving up.

For whatever reason, the word soon got out that I was doing something unusual at my church, and in a short time I was invited to speak in a nearby hall to a new interfaith organization of Catholics, Protestants, and nondenominational believers. I was told that about forty members would be present, but when I arrived more than four hundred people had gathered in the room. I gave a talk on the healing power of God.

After I had finished, the gentleman in charge came over to me and said rather casually that a lot of sick people were in the audience. He asked if I would mind praying for them. I was a parish priest from a very conservative Catholic neighborhood, so I assumed he meant "Pray for these people in the privacy of your home for God's will to be done." That usually meant praying for them to learn to accept their sickness, so I assured him I would be more than happy to do so. But to this man, who was a Pentecostal, prayer and healing meant something much more immediate. He promptly returned to the microphone. "Ron would be delighted to pray for the healing of those in the audience who are sick," he announced happily, "and by so doing to demonstrate the power of God active in our midst. So would anyone interested in healing please come forward now?"

When I heard those words, I almost went into cardiac arrest. Theologically speaking, I believed in the power of God—but the power of God *to heal* was another matter . . . or was it? I sat there stunned as two hundred people began to file up to the podium. That was when I recalled my seminary training, during which one of my professors had told us, "If you're ever caught in a situation where you don't know what to do, look pious." That I could handle. I put my head down and started to count the tiles in the floor, hoping to become not only pious but invisible. The man at the microphone called to me to come over, but he had to walk over to me and literally take me by the arm to get me to go. I had never done anything like a public healing, and I was thinking to myself that I wasn't about to begin now.

My mind was racing to come up with the most pious prayer imaginable. "Now," I said in my best clerical tone of voice, "while every eye is closed and every head is bowed, let us pray." At the same time, I silently uttered to myself the most profoundly theological prayer that came to mind: *Help!*

When you take yourself too seriously, however, the Spirit of God, or what some people might call an angel of the Lord, comes down to touch you and lighten you up—a lesson I learned very well that night. Just at that moment, an astonishing question for a Catholic priest in the early 1970s popped into my mind. I firmly believe that what springs into your mind at moments like these is not at all accidental and I asked myself, What would Oral Roberts do at a time like this?

For the better part of the past year, I had been in the habit of watching Roberts on Sunday morning before going to the church to celebrate mass. Since I knew my congregation probably wouldn't be caught dead watching a Protestant faith healer, I even used to steal some of his sermons! I didn't believe in healing, but the guy was a great preacher and I wasn't above appropriating some of his messages. Now I had use for another of his techniques. I had seen Roberts lay hands on people, so I instantly decided I should emulate him in this as well. With that thought in mind, I walked off the platform toward the woman at the head of the line.

All of a sudden, I was seized with a bad case of second-guessing. Wait a minute, I thought, laying on of hands is what the *Protestants* do! Catholics make the sign of the cross. And in fact, the woman in front of me turned out to be Catholic. "Just bless me, Father," she said. Bless her or lay hands on her, what should I do? Then the voice of God said very loudly to me, "Give her double or nothing!"

I laid my left hand on the woman's forehead and blessed her with my right, as out of my mouth came the words, "You're healed!" And I continued to move swiftly through the crowd, speeding up the process as I went so that I could make a quick exit. I arrived home that night somewhat exhausted by an experience that I had neither desired nor planned and proceeded to put the entire event out of my mind.

Approximately four months later, the woman I had touched at the front of the line showed up on the doorstep of my church to share with me what had happened to her since that healing service. She began by saying that she had never experienced anything like it in her life. "When you touched me," she said, "I felt a lightning bolt go through me. And I heard a voice say to me, 'Go back to your doctor.'"

She then revealed to me for the first time that prior to coming to my talk she had been diagnosed with lung cancer. "On Monday morning, I called my doctor," she continued, "and said I wanted to come in for some more tests."

The day after the tests were done, her doctor informed her that no trace of cancer could be detected.

From the day she told me that story, my life followed a direction I had not consciously charted and could not have predicted.

The focal point of my consciousness shifted from preaching to spiritual healing. People began coming to me for help, although at the time I did not understand how I could provide this help. I was following a meandering path of gradual recognition, with plenty of fits and starts along the way, and my destination was often far from clear. I had begun to hold an ecumenical service on Monday nights at my church because I wanted to meet the needs of Protestants and Catholics who had intermarried and felt excluded from their own churches. One night a woman in a wheelchair was brought to me at the service. I was led to touch her on her hip, and as I did so I heard a crackle of electricity and suddenly the man standing next to her fell to the floor. I was terribly unnerved and said to myself, Thank you, God, but that's enough of this.

After that service, I went back to the rectory with the firm intention of having a long talk with the Lord and setting Him straight. But what I found out is that God talks, we listen. I began to realize that I had little control over what was happening through me other than to make myself the clearest channel I could. Around this time a phrase from the Prayer of Saint Francis embedded itself in my consciousness: "Lord, make me an instrument of your peace." This suggested that I needed to surrender to a force far greater than myself, a force that could be trusted to do the work *through* me. I needed only to offer that "spiritual force" a vehicle through which to operate. Gradually I gave in to God's desire and began to learn how to heal by the power of God's Spirit, which emanates from love and fills the whole universe with its divine energy.

As I continued my healing services, I saw people get out of their wheelchairs or drop their crutches. I received reports from some who were healed of cancer and from women who had been unable to conceive but who were now pregnant—all of these cases verified by their own doctors. In many instances, I did not even have to touch physically the person seeking healing. All that was needed was my intention to be the channel of God's divine energy, no matter what the circumstances.

As a direct result of these experiences, I became convinced that prayer was the conduit of the healing energy that my parishioners and I tangibly felt. On some occasions, I actually experienced a presence; at other times, tremendous heat would fill the church or the sound of electrical discharge would ripple through the air. Since it has always been plain to me that I am perfectly ordinary in almost every way, I knew that I could not be personally responsible for these healings. I continued to ask God for an explanation of what was happening, and one evening I received a very long dissertation that I can briefly summarize: "It is not up to you. You don't need to know what is happening or why. Your job is to pray, to connect, to love and show compassion for people. I do the rest."

I still couldn't help asking what kind of prayer was the key to this startling energy release and the healings that were occurring through me. The kind of prayer I had been taught as a Catholic boy growing up in the Midwest had never had this kind of effect. On reflection, I realized that I had never had a single course on how to pray. Even during my years in the seminary, we had received no instruction on the Lord's Prayer, perhaps the most important prayer in the Christian canon, and we had had no course on invoking the Holy Spirit. When we had studied the sacraments, we focused entirely on getting the ritual correct. We had never talked about whether the sacraments or prayer generated energy of any sort.

Based on my own experiences with prayer after leaving the seminary, however, I had begun to reexamine what I believed and what I had been taught. I gradually came to realize that the essence of genuine prayer lies not in the words themselves or in some attitude of solemnity or piousness but in our focus on God and the attributes of God. As I learned to center myself on God rather than obsessing about my personal difficulties or problems, prayers like the Our Father and the 23rd Psalm, which had grown stale and devoid of energy from years of perfunctory recitation, began to come alive in me. God began to reveal Himself as a genuine presence, a living, vibrating energy.

At the time, I hadn't heard of "centering prayer," a method of meditative prayer promulgated in the 1970s and '80s by Father Thomas Keating, a Cistercian monk and the former abbot of St. Joseph's Abbey in Spencer, Massachusetts, and Father Basil Pennington, a Trappist monk also at St. Joseph's. Centering prayer combined early Christian mystical models, especially the anonymous fourteenth-century treatise *The Cloud of Unknowing*, and certain Eastern techniques, most notably the Transcendental Meditation developed by Maharishi Mahesh Yogi.

I had stumbled across my own version of centering prayer, which I deepened by readings of the Desert Fathers and medieval Christian mystical works, including *The Cloud*. I may not have called it centering prayer back then, but that would have been the right name for what I had begun to do: centering on the core of who I really was. I began to simplify my prayers, letting myself dwell on a single word or phrase until the repetition carried me into a blissful feeling of unity with God unlike any I had achieved from wordier prayers. The principles of this kind of prayer are quite simple and can be easily learned by anyone willing to try.

1. Begin by choosing a sacred word that is a symbol of your intention to consent to the presence and action of God within you. The word could be the name of Jesus in English, Greek, or Aramaic, for instance, or the name of any sacred Being or holy person of your choice, like the Buddha, Kuan Yin, or Sri Ramakrishna. Or it could be a word such as "love,"

"peace," or "surrender," or an attribute of God such as "mercy" or "light."

2. Silently introduce the sacred word into your awareness, reminding yourself that you are using this word as a symbol of your intention to consent to God's presence and action in your life.

3. When distractions come to you—and they will—gently return to the sacred word and continue to repeat it to yourself.

The beauty of this kind of prayer is that you can do it at any time and any place—at your desk in the office, on the bus, in bed before going to sleep. In fact, as we will see in subsequent chapters, learning ways to maintain your connection with God throughout the day is in itself one of the keys to prayer as a healing path.

You are probably familiar with some variation of the saying, "As you think, so shall you be." The earliest version of this saying that I'm aware of appears at the opening of the Dhammapada, or sayings of the Buddha, reaching back over 2,500 years. By placing sacred names or the attributes of God in your consciousness continually, you begin to absorb them into your very being. You become "centered" on God and His attributes. But don't be discouraged if this doesn't seem to happen the moment you begin praying this way. The path is strewn with obstacles, as I can attest.

After praying in this manner for some years, I suddenly realized for the first time in my life the major role that fear plays in our spiritual life. I had always suspected that my prayers were *not* being answered instead of assuming that they were or would be. I would pray, but assume—or fear—that a problem would not go away. My worry and fear about the problem would actually block my perception of the problem and of any God-given resolution to it!

Our fears short-circuit the energy emitted during our

communion with God. No wonder the Old and New Testaments contain so many imperatives to "fear not." By some scholars' estimation, the Bible has 365 references to being fearless. ("Fear not, I am with you," the Lord says to the prophet Isaiah. In the Gospels of Luke and Matthew, Mary and Joseph are both told by an angel of God not to be afraid.)

Spoken with my new awareness, however, the words of the Lord's Prayer and the 23rd Psalm now held a vibrational energy that dissipated my fears, at least temporarily. There was no doubt in my mind. I felt the strength that filled the absence of fear! Since fear is the major block to receiving healing energy, I knew I had to reshape my spiritual healing work with an emphasis on teaching people to "fear not." I was further motivated and determined to do this when I recalled how a young woman had come to one of my healing meetings, propped up by two canes. I caught a glimpse of her as she arrived late to the meeting, very unsteady and hardly able to walk. She didn't come forward for personal prayer at the conclusion of the meeting, but she did return the following week. On that night, she came forward for personal prayer. I was moved to do something I had never done before. I gently pulled the canes away from her, touched her forehead with one finger, and urged her to "walk." She crumpled to the floor and lay there for the next twenty minutes. Then she slowly got to her feet and began walking perfectly.

Some time later this woman came to me privately and told me her sad story. Both her husband and her children were abusive to her. She had been so consumed by the fear of falling that she had not left her home for the past three years. The terror she experienced daily had begun to cripple every part of her being, until the night she attended the healing meeting.

During the next few years, her regular attendance at our church was a source of constant amazement to people who had known the woman in her previous condition. She was able to come and go as she pleased without any need for her canes. At the same time, she found the strength to stand up to her family and tell them she wasn't going to take it anymore. They backed off, and she seemed to get her life on track. Then, for reasons that I never learned, she stopped showing up at services. I subsequently heard that she had once again given in to the abusive relationship. She had also, not coincidentally, returned to being an invalid and being invalidated by fear. The last I heard, she had completely reverted to staying at home and walking with canes.

By way of contrast, let me tell you the story of a young woman who came to a healing mass in 1991, when I was still a parish priest. Three and a half years before, following a miscarriage and subsequent treatment with an experimental antidepressant drug, she had again become pregnant. During a routine sonogram in the fifth month of her pregnancy, the technicians discovered two small masses in her uterine wall, which her obstetrician diagnosed as benign fibroid tumors. She eventually bore a healthy baby boy, and was told not to worry about the fibroid masses that were still present. When the masses continued to grow, a biopsy showed that they were in fact cancerous. New tumors had also appeared, and the woman's doctors insisted on immediate surgery to remove the tumors. She was already under tremendous stress from a failing marriage and the ensuing financial crisis that threatened foreclosure of her home.

Despite the warnings from her doctors, including their suggestion that she make a will, the woman put off surgery for several months. In January 1991, as she later informed me in a letter, she was "talked into" attending a healing mass I was celebrating. "I did not believe in such nonsense," she wrote, "plus I did not feel up to attending. In the end I went only because the women in my mother's group had insisted."

Nevertheless, when I asked for anyone at that healing mass

who was in physical pain to stand up and place their hands where the pain was, she did so. As I prayed over the congregation, her letter stated, "The pain literally washed away. It felt like someone had poured water over my head, and as it passed over my body it took the pain with it."

The woman subsequently attended another healing session with her grandmother. "I figured maybe, just maybe . . ." she wrote. One month later, she returned to her doctors for a scheduled sonogram and the much-delayed surgery. The technician who read the sonogram, however, could find no tumors. Although the woman had tried to tell her doctors about the healing services, they hadn't really listened. And now they were too busy second-guessing each other. Rechecking the original sonogram, they were reassured to see clear evidence of the tumors but didn't know what to make of the new images. Still arguing loudly with each other, the doctors scheduled surgery to do a "look see." The operation revealed scar tissue growth but no tumors. Not taking any chances, they cleared the uterus with a laser, which was likely to leave the woman sterile.

Three months later she was feeling unwell and came back to her doctors, thinking that the tumors might have returned. This time the sonogram revealed no tumors but a perfectly normal six-week-old fetus. "Life has taken on a whole new meaning," she wrote to me. "I still get confused but life is a lot easier to get back on track."

Faith grows in the least expected places. This woman came to a healing service against her better judgment, yet faith took root and flourished through some difficult situations, proving the words of Jesus that whoever "does not doubt in his heart, but believes that what he says will come to pass, it will be done for him." She was able to transcend her doubts and take hold of the healing that she had been given.

The story of the first woman, who fell back into her abusive relationship, shows that we have to be involved in our own healing. Without being receptive to God's energy, we cannot genuinely heal. Unless we nourish that receptivity daily and keep it active within us, as the second woman did, a healing can even revert to illness. So when you pray, be aware of whether you are listening to God or just bombarding Him with requests. If the words "Lord, help me . . ." appear frequently in your prayers, stop a moment and see if you can turn your requests into affirmations: "Lord, I know you give me strength to face the difficulties of this day. You inspire me with the wisdom to come up with creative solutions to any dilemma."

Moreover, when we pray for healing we must also acknowledge our own thoughts and feelings. Acknowledging and owning our thoughts and feelings isn't the same as obsessing about them, as I had been doing before I began centering on God. Focusing can clearly be positive or negative; obsessing about, say, chronic financial difficulties and complaining to God about a lack of money is different from focusing on the problem in a positive way. You might, for instance, pray: "I know, Lord, that your desire is to prosper me in all areas of my life. Right now I open my entire being to receive your prosperity flow." That's not just an idle affirmation or wishful thinking, but is based on a sacred truth that God wants us to live abundantly. Rather than fighting the problem head-on, you replace the negativity with an expression that is positive. In effect, you learn to pray differently, as I will discuss in much greater depth in Chapter 4 on the Lord's Prayer.

Acknowledging our deepest thoughts and feelings is not always easy, because we may have hidden agendas that tend to obscure self-knowledge. I recently received a letter from a woman who had attended one of my workshops and had approached me afterward to ask if I could help her friend, who was experiencing a great deal of pain. "People are truly funny," the woman wrote, "and

I guess that it is true that we sometimes do not want to heal. [My friend] was so angry at you because all of her pain went away, and now she was afraid that she would have to go off workman's comp and go back to work. So, needless to say, she created more problems once we arrived home. We had a wonderful trip home and we were laughing with her because she felt great. And then the fear came in. . . ."

If an issue is blocking your healing, God will work on it in two ways, as I explain in my workshops. One way God does this is by bringing the issue to the surface consciously when you open yourself to Him during prayer. The other way is what I would call the resting of the spirit element, which may occur when an issue might be too much for you to bear on a conscious level. As you are being prayed for or with by me or by others in a healing workshop, let's say, you may go to sleep or into a trancelike state and stay there for as long as an hour. That usually indicates that something is being healed on a very deep level that would be too painful for you to be consciously aware of at the time. If you need to remember it down the road because it is blocking your moving forward and becoming whole, it will come back to your conscious memory at that point, but the sting will have been removed.

Healing, then, involves the whole self: body, mind, emotions, and spirit. To bring your whole self into prayer, first see yourself and others as spirit, a being whose soul happens to be, at this time, encased in a body. You are not just your body any more than you are just your mind; you are spirit. Practice seeing others as spirits in bodies, too.

For our spirit to be continually nourished, we need to make room for it, acknowledge it, feed it through prayer and reflective moments in our daily lives. Prayer and meditation reconnect us with God, the Life Force of our being. To pray is to be spiritually treated by the medicine of God—His divine energy. I will help you pray effectively, in a way that taps that divine energy, if you think of the nature of God as light-energy.

Meditation on Transformation into the Light-Energy of God

All the prayers and meditations in this book are simple exercises to release the energy of God within you so you can be strengthened and begin to heal. The more we center on the presence of God that fills the world around us and every part of our being, and the more we commune with God in this manner, the more we become aware of the almighty energy that restores, revives, and heals. Everyone becomes a little depleted at times during the day. We tend to blame the people around us, especially our boss, or spouse, or children. You don't have to blame anyone. Go off for a minute and get reenergized by doing any one of these exercises. God will energize you if you just make the connection.

When I speak of God throughout these exercises, I am asking you to evoke whatever image and sense of God is meaningful to you. As pure Spirit that encompasses all existence, God has no sex, although for convenience I still often use the masculine pronoun. You may prefer to conceptualize God as female, or in any of the myriad concrete images that have been used to represent the Absolute throughout history and around the globe. Indeed, humankind seems to need personal images of both sexes to render accessible that most inconceivable Being. Although Buddhists eschew the concept of a Supreme Being, for instance, they revere numerous images of buddhas, bodhisattvas, and dakinis, male and female, earthly and celestial, and use them extensively to focus their spiritual energies. The image or conceptualization you use is of significance mainly to you.

If you are not in the habit of focusing on spiritual images, I recommend that you take some time to find one that you are comfortable with. Begin with your birth religion, even if you have not practiced it actively for some time. And don't limit yourself to the most obvious images or only to images of God or the Absolute. If you come from a Christian background, the most familiar images are of Jesus and Mother Mary. Yet many others are available to you, including personifications of Mary as the patron saint of various ethnic groups—from Our Lady of Czestochowa (Poland) to Our Lady of Guadalupe (Mexico). Literally hundreds of saints and mystics of both sexes are also available, and images of many of them can be purchased in any good religious supply store. Even the Jewish and Islamic traditions, which do not allow the use of images of the Almighty, do use visual representations drawn from Hebrew and Arabic calligraphy to focus their energy.

You may feel more at ease, however, with images from the various Eastern traditions or Native American spirituality, which don't carry for you the weight of oppressive childhood religious training. Throughout these meditations and exercises, you may want to substitute the most common embodiments of the sacred drawn from those traditions—such as Shiva, Kali, Kuan Yin, Tara, Chenrezi, the Buddha, and the Great Spirit of the American Indians, called Wakan Tanka by the Lakota Sioux—or some of the great saints and sages known for their wisdom and compassion. Mirabai, Ramana Maharshi, Sri Ramakrishna, and Anandamayi Ma from India, Milarepa and the Dalai Lama from Tibet, and Buffalo Calf Woman of the North American Indians are all appropriate figures whose images can be found in books.

You may also choose to visualize one of the many current teachers to whose talks or writings you have responded, remaining cognizant that a number of these teachers have been touched by controversy. Without necessarily agreeing or disagreeing with the charges that have been leveled at a surprising number of modern-day teachers, try to keep your heart open to the possibility that perfectly valid and helpful teachings can come through flawed vessels of transmission, just as great works of art have been created by masters whose attitudes about race and sexual stereotypes might not seem enlightened by current standards. Even Mother Teresa has not escaped being accused of inappropriate activity. Accusations of the most odious behavior against the late Cardinal Joseph Bernardin were ultimately retracted by his accuser. I often think of Cardinal Bernardin in my prayers. Although he clearly suffered greatly at being publicly defamed, he treated his accuser with enormous compassion and tenderness both before and after the man recanted. In the final months of Cardinal Bernardin's life, as he himself was dying of cancer, this holy man visited with other sick and dying people in the Chicago area and taught us all a great lesson in dying with dignity and a kind of selfless detachment. Few historical figures carry for me the kind of inspirational energy that the Cardinal holds.

Finally, although it may be easiest to perform these exercises in private, some of you may wish to join with a spouse or partner, with your children, or with a small group of friends. I will address some of these exercises and rituals to both individual and group use where appropriate. In particular, some of the sacramental rituals that I have reconceptualized in Chapter 9 lend themselves to group celebration. You may even want to prerecord the meditations on an audiocassette for your own use or for group prayer.

MEDITATION

Now, to begin our first exercise, take three deep breaths and release yourself from the thoughts and concerns of your day. Breathing normally, spend a few minutes just following your own breath as a way of grounding yourself, observing where your breath flows into and out of your body, and any feelings or sensations associated with it. When you have settled in, begin to envision or sense a glowing light surrounding your heart. See that light as the very presence of God, the very energy of God that emanates from the love and mercy of God. Love and mercy is the very personality of God that makes God all-powerful. Envision and sense that merciful and loving light now moving through every part of your body: your shoulders, your arms, your hands, your torso, your legs, your feet, your eyes, your ears, your throat, the crown of your head, until your whole body is engulfed in light. As your body is being flooded with light, you are being engulfed by the energy that is the mercy and love of God.

Imagine a powerful ray of light moving from the center of your body to the top of your head and out of your body. If you are doing this exercise in a group, imagine that your ray meets all of the other lights in the room until they converge into one ocean of light. You are now swimming in the very presence of God, whose Spirit is everywhere, whose energy is everywhere. Now allow the Spirit of God to call to mind someone in need of this ray of energy that you have released through prayer. Usually the Holy Spirit will simply impress a name or face upon your mind or thought. Just allow that light to leave the room instantly and surround and fill the person of whom you are thinking. Do this in silence, because numerous names or faces may come to you. In the next few moments, allow the Holy Spirit of God, the breath of life, or prana, if you prefer that term, to move and encase others. As you are projecting or allowing this light to move from you, see what it is also doing *to* you. Feel the energy that is coming to you.

As you give, you receive. So whether you are working or engaged in recreation, socializing, or doing housework by yourself, you can stop for a moment and allow the Spirit to fill you with light. Then allow that Spirit to bring to your mind those you can pray for. Pray for them simply by relaxing and allowing the Spirit to release itself in an instant—for there are no boundaries of time or space in the world of the spiritual. In that instant, surround that person with love, peace, and the presence of God, which is light.

Do this simply because you desire that other person's wholeness and health. Then the Holy Spirit will draw that time to a close.

Maybe a few other times throughout the day, the Spirit of God, the voice of God—what we might call a hunch or idea—will come to you. At that moment, stop and allow yourself to be what you truly are: light. Allow that light, that presence of God, to move out of you, and as it energizes and heals others it returns to you. When you are done, take three deep breaths and begin to open your eyes.

T W O

GOD IS LIGHT-ENERGY

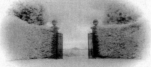

"Let there be light! And there was light" (Gen. 1:3). In the creation of the universe, God's first command brought into being the structural essential: light. On the beams of this immaterial medium occur all divine manifestations. Devotees of every age testify to the appearance of God as flame and light. "His eyes were as a flame of fire," Saint John tells us, ". . . and his countenance was as the sun shineth in his strength" (Rev. 1:14–16).

◆

PARAMAHANSA YOGANANDA, *AUTOBIOGRAPHY OF A YOGI*

All things that are, are light.

◆

EZRA POUND

According to the famous opening verses of the first chapter of Genesis, "In the beginning God created the heavens and the earth. The earth was formless and empty, and darkness was upon the face of the deep; and the Spirit of God was moving over the face of the waters. And God said, 'Let there be light'; and there was light" (Gen. 1:1–3).

What is implied in this passage? God first decides to create. A blueprint or plan exists in the mind of God, the Creator. The Creator then speaks and the word goes forth to begin the act of creating the universe over the course of time. Form takes place out of formlessness, when God says, "Let there be . . ." The Creator speaks the word and the whole process of creation begins. God creates "light" first, bringing into existence that which would be the essence of all life: light-energy.

The essence of God is light; the essence of God is energy. So when God said, "Let there be light," He created from the essence of His own being and set into motion a process in which everything created from this time on would contain the essence and the life of God. Through the spoken word, energy was created. Everything created from that point on was created out of light, out of energy, the primal energy I call "Holy Spirit," which was there at the beginning of creation according to the Genesis account. Vibrations of power emanated from the spoken word of God and are eternally present, emanating from the essence of God because energy never dies. Through the flow of creative energy, everything else came into being in an orderly fashion.

I find it interesting that the next element God created was water, since water is one of the great conductors of electricity. Following this came the creation of the land, plants, and trees. On the fourth day, the denseness began to clear as the stars and all the other planetary objects that God created became visible. Only then did He create the sun and the moon. Clearly His initial command for there to be light had nothing to do with what we normally associate with the light of the sun or the reflected light of the moon.

Living creatures then evolved, beginning with those that inhabited the water. After the fish came into being, all other living creatures, including man and woman, were fashioned. Upon completion, God gave a command to the humans stating they were to increase and be the masters—or stewards—of all other life on the planet. In other words, we who are made in God's likeness—that is, light and energy—are to create as God creates. The same primal energy that designed the universe in the beginning is still at work with us and in us to help continue our work in the plan of cocreation.

Knowing God as an experienced reality is the crux of spiritual healing. We have just seen how God is light. In the Bible, the reality of God is often referred to as "fire," which is another form of energy. To experience the fire energy of God, we need to know first off that the nature of God is spirit. We also need to realize that, having been made in the image of God, we too are spirit; to know God, then, we must return to our essential nature as spirit.

Many fundamentalist Christians are fond of using the term "born again" without understanding what it really means. For me, being born again refers to a rebirth of self-worth. Fire can be a powerful symbol for the rebirthing process because just as fire consumes matter, the fire of God consumes our ego-nature, producing only ashes. Into the ashes a new life is breathed, which represents the action of the Holy Spirit of God making us aware of our true essence as spirit. Through that awareness, we are authentically "born again" and given the opportunity to grow in the nature of God, from whom we have come. We mature through our development of God-consciousness, a consciousness born of our communion with the Creator.

When using prayer as spiritual-energy medicine, we would be wise to view how this energy was released in former times, for example, by Solomon, Jesus, and the followers of Jesus. Whether it was released to heal, cure, multiply the loaves and fishes, or bring God's fire into the Temple is not the issue. Our primary concern is in discovering what caused that energy to be released.

Some type of divine energy is physically manifested when the Holy Spirit of God is released upon an individual or a group of people. In Chapters 6 and 7 of the Old Testament book known as 2nd Chronicles, we get a vibrant picture of the presence of God manifesting as a consuming energy so powerful that people fall to the ground during an intensive time of prayer. After Solomon completed the building of the Temple, the Ark of the Covenant was carried into the inner sanctuary, its final resting place. "All the Levites who were musicians stood on the east side of the altar dressed in fine linen, playing their instruments," the text reads. "They were accompanied by 120 priests sounding trumpets. The trumpeters and singers joined in one accord, with one voice to give thanks and praise to God."

This, then, was their ritual prayer: "His loving kindness endures forever." Simple and to the point! After this the Temple of God was filled with a cloud. The Holy Spirit filled the area like a mist, just as the mist comes in over the ocean in the evenings. When I have sat on the shore watching the mist approaching, I have felt as though it were going right through me, just like the awesome presence of Spirit in this episode.

The cloud that filled the Temple of the Lord was so thick it hindered the priests from performing their service. Then Solomon began to pray a marvelous prayer of forgiveness, in which he repeated the phrase "Forgive your people, O Lord." In effect, he was asking God to release the Israelites from the boomerang effects of their negative way of living. In the name of the people gathered together, Solomon connected with God through a series of declarations, petitions, affirmations, and statements of forgiveness, culminating in the invitation "And now arise, O Lord God, and go to your resting place" (6:41).

"When Solomon had ended his prayer," we are told at the beginning of Chapter 7, "fire came down from heaven and consumed the burnt offerings and the sacrifices, and the glory of the Lord filled the temple." Solomon used several of the basic forms of communion with God known as prayer and, as a result, the presence and power of God was manifested.

To connect with God's fire and healing energy, the people of Israel in this text used as their prayer the words of Psalm 136: "The Lord is Good. His loving kindness endures forever." This prayer was often used by the Israelites in their communion with God. You too can repeat this affirmation frequently until you sense the fire of God welling up within you. When the Israelites affirmed these words concerning God's goodness upon entering the temple with the Ark of the Covenant, God's glory filled the place with His light. Take three minutes right now to repeat this prayer slowly and quietly to yourself at least ten times, but more if you feel so moved.

In the New Testament book of Acts, the disciples of Jesus focused their attention on God for ten days as Jesus taught them to do in the Lord's Prayer. At the culmination of these ten days, they experienced something marvelous. Flames appeared along with a blowing wind, whereupon they discovered they could heal the sick and speak in languages they had never learned. They had encountered the Spirit of God as living energy.

As we can see from these stories, connecting with God is the primary activator in releasing the fire and energy of God. This is especially true in any large gathering of people as depicted in 2nd Chronicles. The spiritual leader, like Solomon, acts as a conduit to release God's energy for healing. The spiritual leader brings the people into oneness with God and one another through prayer just as Solomon did.

Like Solomon, spiritual leaders such as Kathryn Kuhlman and Aimee Semple McPherson were effective healers in the twentieth century largely because of their ability to focus on God and get others to do the same. They acted as conduits for the attention of the people, gathering it to them and redirecting that focus onto the omnipotent God, whose spiritual energy was then channeled back to the people via the spiritual leader. High-voltage energy can be released in such groups of people. Taking my cue from Kuhlman and McPherson, I have used music in conjunction with prayer to bring people at my gatherings into harmony within themselves and with each other. Even thousands of people can feel united by the energy of love and joy without the emotional hype or manipulation that many so-called faith healers contrive.

At one such event I was asked to conduct a call to prayer for twelve thousand people. As the soft music of "Amazing Grace" echoed in the background, I felt as if I were filled with words from another dimension. No sooner had those words flowed from my lips than a rush of energy suddenly punctuated the assembly. Lines of people slowly began to make their way to the front of the auditorium where I was standing, some leaving their empty wheelchairs on the stage area, others placing their hearing aids in the hands of my staff, while many in the audience were sobbing. I was stunned. There was no doubt in my mind that this was a visit from the Creator, the Healer, the Lover of all mankind. We were touching and being touched by the fire and energy of God that is the Holy Spirit.

God's power had punctuated the atmosphere, reminding me

of that first Pentecost described in the Book of Acts. This event speaks of a fire entering the room where the disciples were in one accord (harmony), praying. The "fire" penetrated their very beings, healing them of their fears, empowering them to embark on an adventure of great spiritual magnitude. That fire is still available, waiting for us to take hold of it and embark on our own adventure of spiritual truth.

Whatever the scientific definition of electricity may be, most of us associate it with its manifestation as light and heat. If God is light energy that sometimes manifests as fire, it's not a stretch of the imagination to see God as electrical energy. But we can also look at electricity in ways other than as a manifestation of light and heat. It is in the air all the time, just as are broadcast waves covering a wide range of frequencies. Electricity may manifest as a voice over a telephone or as paper rolling off a fax machine, provided the phone and fax are switched on and ready to receive. With the help of electricity, broadcast waves manifest as pictures on a television set or as radio programs or short-wave communications, provided our receivers are turned on and tuned in.

These energies are always present in the atmosphere, but they become palpable for us only when we set our appropriate receivers to catch them. Anyone who has ever had a problem with TV or radio reception, or with getting a phone line or a fax machine to work properly, knows that tuning properly to receive the transmission isn't always as easy as it seems. I feel the same way about prayer. Divine energy is in the atmosphere surrounding us all the time, but unless our receiver is turned on and properly tuned, we may not be able to avail ourselves of it.

Part of the problem is that although we are the receivers of divine energy, we often act as if we were the transmitters. When we pray, we are constantly babbling to God about what we need and what we want for ourselves and others instead of listening for God's message to us. Although it is not wrong to ask God for help for others who are suffering, we have to know how to do this in the proper spirit. Much has been said and written about the value of intercessory prayer, but unfortunately most people don't have a clear understanding of what it actually is.

Intercessory prayer has nothing to do with words. To pray, for example, "Dear God, please heal my mother, who is suffering from ovarian cancer," is not especially effective. The key to true intercessory prayer is compassion. Genuine compassion—a word that comes from Latin roots meaning literally "to bear or suffer with"—isn't easily developed. Suffering in your own life may teach you what it feels like to be in the position of someone who is ill, or in emotional distress, or homeless, but we are called on to empathize with many people and we will never experience all possible forms of distress. The best way to develop compassion is through the discipline of daily prayer and meditation.

How do we do this? Begin by trying to put yourself in the position of the person for whom you are praying. What does it feel like to be told by the doctor that you have an inoperable brain tumor and that you have only six months to live? How does it feel to learn that your child has just been killed or maimed in an automobile accident, or that a loved one has committed suicide? Every day before you begin to pray, put yourself in the position of the person for whom you are praying. You may never have had his or her experiences, or you may have prayed that such things never happen to you. In a sense, other people's experiences also happen to us through the connection of our common spiritual natures and energy. To pray effectively, we need to reexperience feelings that we have blocked out. When I pray for the healing of others, I write their names on a piece of paper and then I open myself to what they may be feeling, whether it is fear, anxiety, or physical pain. As John Donne said in those lines that people often quote without knowing what they actually mean, "Each man's death diminishes me, for I am involved in mankind." All of those things you most fear have *already* happened to you because they have happened to other human beings to whom you are intimately connected.

Spend a few moments asking God to let you feel what the person for whom you are praying feels. God will then make a strong heart connection between you and that person. At that point it doesn't matter exactly what you say: "Lord, heal him now. Help her now. Remove their fears now. Give her a sense of your peace now. Clear his body of this cancer now, Lord, with your love." Your heart will give you the words when you've made the connection.

Intercessory prayer, then, really means standing in for another and assuming that he or she doesn't know how to pray, or can't pray, or is not praying for one reason or another. After placing yourself in this person's place, you may wait for instructions from God about how to approach this particular problem. All prayer is the reception of the light energy that is the presence of God. It may take the form of guidance, prophecy, wisdom, clairvoyance, or even a simple hunch or gut feeling or spontaneous idea.

Receiving the energy is only part of the process. We also have to act on the messages we receive from God, whether they are for another or for ourselves. What we must do after prayer is act in congruency with what we have just received. Take, for example, the message I received as a child: "Touch your hands to your throat and you will be healed." I acted as if it were true because I believed and trusted that voice, but if I hadn't trusted it and hadn't acted, I don't believe I would have been healed in that fashion. I might have survived and been cured somehow through medical intervention, but that might have had other consequences that I'll never know.

Most of the time we're not even open to hearing the voice of our own intuitions. When I was a parish priest, I suffered from a problem in my feet that made it painful for me to stand up. This condition had persisted for months, but I had steadfastly ignored my intuition to seek a spiritual healing for myself. Maybe I thought I wasn't worthy. One Sunday while I was saying mass, I felt I could no longer tolerate the pain and I finally became desperate enough to listen to the voice that came to me just prior to the consecration of the host. "This time," the voice said, "look at the host as truly being light that heals. Visualize the wine in the cup as shimmering, supernatural light, the light of God's energy." I was to allow the picture to come into my mind of this light-energy traveling from my mouth throughout my entire body, down to my feet. Listening to this inner voice, I entertained the possibility that this supernatural light-energy, taken internally through drinking the wine, could heal me. My conscious mind ought to have fought that notion, but perhaps I was in so much pain that I was willing to listen and accept it. Upon consuming the wine, I felt an exhilaration of peace and love. By the end of the communion service, I was able to stand more comfortably, and by the time I returned to the rectory the pain in my feet had completely disappeared. I've had other physical maladies since, but that particular problem has never returned.

Spiritual electricity surrounds us in many different forms. In the first letter of John is the declaration "God is love." But that epistle begins by stating, "This is the message we have heard from Him and proclaim to you, that God is light, and in Him is no darkness at all" (1:5). Saint James in his epistle says, "Every good gift comes down from the Father of lights" (1:17). These scriptures convince me that when we are connected with the Source, which is Light, what is coming to us is undoubtedly light. Paul says, "Now you are light in the Lord; walk as children of light" (Eph. 5:8). People take that as metaphor, but it's not; it's reality.

These statements closely resemble Hindu teachings. The great mystics of all religions have said that when they meditate and touch reality, they see essentially the same thing: light. Light is energy and energy is electricity. A manifestation of that light comes through my body in a healing. There is no difference in mystical terms between the true born-again experience—the fire of Pentecost—and the experience of Kundalini, in which the primal power that lies coiled like a serpent at the base of the spine rises up and sends light shooting out through the crown of the head. Both experiences are awakening stages in which you are in touch with your true Source. What you do with that awareness afterward is where free will comes in.

A HEALING MEDITATION: GOD IS LIGHT

In the first letter of John are three powerful words: "God is light." The light of God that radiated through Jesus is in each of us. As you ponder the words "God is light," bring your awareness to your breathing, because the breath is also a reminder of the very life of God entering into your whole being. As we breathe in, we breathe in the light and the breath of God. As we exhale, that light which has now coursed through our body exits to touch the world around us.

"God is light." Focus on the stillness that this phrase provides. Let the Holy Spirit take over guiding you to the deep revelation of this truth, "God is light." Let the truth speak to your heart and your mind. Allow the Spirit's energy to heal you.

Visualize God's love as light.

I am led to commune with God for your healing, dear reader. In a spirit of thankfulness and gratitude, I pour out this expression of love for you. I see myself embraced by the Christ, filled with the light and energy that raised the human Jesus from the dead. Glory is radiating from my being. Strength and joy well up within me and encase me in a silken wrapping of peace. Having paused for a few moments before continuing to write, I feel overwhelmed by the sweet yet strong presence of love—unconditional love—which God has for all of His creation and children.

Thank you, Lord, for your light, your love, your peace, your presence, which fills and heals the whole world. We are all one in your love and so we all can experience your healing touch upon our lives. Thank you, God.

Now remain quiet for two or three minutes as you let God love you. Through His love, mercy, and compassion, you are going to experience healing as well as the freedom of the sons and daughters of God.

MEDITATION TO SEE YOURSELF AS SPIRIT

This exercise is especially effective when performed in a group setting, but may of course be done alone. If you want to, you may dim the lights because you may have an experience during which you will see light. Some of you will not, but that is not what is important. It's not the experience you have but your receptivity to the experience that matters.

To begin your meditation, seek the guidance of that element of God called the Holy Spirit by saying, "Do with me what you will. Show me how I can better serve my brothers and sisters." Make this time of communion an expression of your desire to grow spiritually. Allow yourself to let go of any fear of God or what God may reveal to you. God will look at your heart, not what flows out of your mouth. Repeat the above invocation for just thirty seconds or so the first time. Work up to ten or twenty minutes or an hour if this proves effective for you.

If you do this exercise with a group of people, take the hand of the person next to you. Alone or together, say, "Come, Spirit of God. Come, reveal your presence, Spirit of the living God. Flow. We are receptive. We welcome you. Let your energy flow."

Now take three deep breaths and prepare for another step up the ladder of consciousness. Ask the Spirit of God to recall the previous meditation exercise in which you saw your whole body filled with light. Return to that state either to see it or sense it to the best of your ability. Don't struggle, but ask for the guidance, for the energy, presence, and wisdom of God to have this occur. When you see yourself as spirit and light filled with the grace and life of God, be aware of how you feel. What's happening in your body? You may feel parts of your body that were tense now begin to relax. You may feel a peace begin to creep slowly into your awareness. Whatever you do feel is not as important right now as the practice of the discipline of awareness.

Sometimes it helps if you take a few more breaths and with each breath be more aware. Ask, Is my body relaxing? Am I experiencing the peace of God, the presence of God? Take some time to do that now. If there is still some tension in your body or you are feeling a little restless, ask yourself, Am I being receptive to the light energy of God?

Breathe in and out three more times, deeply and slowly. If you are still feeling a little tense and restless, or if there is a pain in your body, ask, Do I know myself as spirit, made in the image of God? Be aware now of any answers you are getting, any feelings in your body, any guidance. Sometimes we tend to think this guidance is farfetched. At this point, just be aware of any thoughts or feelings in your body or in the atmosphere around you. Then ask yourself this closing question: Can I be of assistance to God as a channel through which the Spirit of life may be given expression?

After remaining open for a response from the Spirit, thank God for your life at this moment, exactly as it is, and for whatever is occurring in your life. After that short time of gratitude, you may begin slowly to open your eyes. Be aware. That is your practice today: the discipline of awareness. You may want to close by affirming to yourself that God is a good God. God is pure goodness, and nothing that emanates from God is anything but good.

THREE

PRAYER WITHOUT CEASING

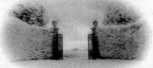

When you are praying in God's presence, examine yourself honestly,
speak to Him if you can; if you can't, stay there, let Him look at you
and don't do anything else.

◆

PADRE PIO

Throughout my twenty-five-year search for authentic Christianity as taught by Jesus, I have discovered that prayer is not a matter of doing but of being. The key to experiencing authentic prayer as taught by the holy ones of all religions is being receptive. In the Book of Acts, the Apostles prayed that the people would *receive* the Holy Spirit. Being receptive means being open to receive the light-energy of God; but to be filled up with God, we must first empty ourselves. In the resulting state of receptivity, we realize the wisdom, counsel, health, provision, and all that is needed in life.

In the Old Testament story of Samuel, the prophet lived in the Temple as a young boy (1 Sam. 3). One night at the age of twelve as he prepared to sleep, he heard a voice speak to him. The voice simply called out, "Samuel! Samuel!" Samuel ran all over the Temple seeking to discover who was calling his name. After this had happened a number of times, he finally asked his teacher, Eli, for help. The teacher told Samuel that when he heard the voice again, he should respond to it by saying, "Here I am, Lord. Your servant is listening." That same voice of God calls each of us today. But if we don't understand authentic prayer as communion with God in a state of receptivity, we will never hear that still small voice within.

The word for prayer in Aramaic, the language Jesus spoke, is *slotha,* the root of which means literally "to set a trap." In the sense in which Jesus used the term, he meant that when we pray we should keep our attention focused and wait patiently to catch the thoughts God has for us. This is equivalent to the receptivity of Christian mystics like Saint Francis, whose famous prayer begins "Lord, make me an instrument of your peace." It may also be akin to the Buddhist concept of *shunyata,* which is usually translated as "emptiness," but might better be rendered as "transparency" or "openness." Christ's conception of praying was the opposite of what prayer has come to mean: begging God for help or special favors. The attitude Jesus advocated in prayer was one of being completely open to whatever thoughts, feelings, or desires God wants to convey to us.

With that in mind, when you pray you might say, "I am receptive to whatever you want to do or give me, God. It will be enough for today." Edgar Cayce repeatedly told people to pray in that very manner: "God, do with me what you will." All the mystics prayed that kind of prayer, which may sound scary at first. If you are convinced that God is just waiting to hear you acknowledge your openness to His divine will so you can be made to *suffer*, you may hesitate to offer yourself to Him in this fashion. Yet I don't believe that God intends for us to suffer or be sick. Oftentimes, we can bring suffering and sickness on ourselves, but His intention is for us to be healthy.

The third chapter of the Book of Proverbs reminds us to acknowledge God in all we do. For years, I didn't have the faintest idea of what that meant. I thought that to say, "Jesus, Jesus, Jesus" would be acknowledging God. If I just begged or pleaded with God, I thought that would be acknowledging Him. I learned through trial and error that to acknowledge God I had to sit in God's presence to perceive the world as God perceives it—as spirit, light, energy. Everything else is illusion. This is what religionists call the carnal mind, by which they mean perceiving reality as matter. (The carnal mind does not mean "sins of the flesh.") All the world's mystics have said, in essence, that until we realize that everything is light, or spirit, we won't really progress on the spiritual path. They do not mean that we should not honor matter, especially the body, because that is where we are right now. Devaluing the body and matter, as Christianity has all too often tended to do, desensitizes us to human suffering and ultimately leads us to an easy acceptance of social ills from pollution to murder. Acknowledging God requires that we strike a balance between seeing the world as spirit and honoring the material forms that spirit has taken on. Swami Muktananda, the Indian master of Siddha Yoga who taught in this country in the 1970s and '80s, put it this way in his book *Play of Consciousness:*

> If God were not in the world, who could live there? Who would strive to make his worldly dealings honest and pure? If the world is interesting and full of joy, it is because of God. . . . It is only because the bliss of the supremely blissful Lord is reflected in the world that we derive a little satisfaction from all sense pleasures and from all worldly actions. We find the shadow of God's bliss in the taste of food, in the sweetness of water, in the melodies of the *ragas* and *raginis,* in the soft smile of blossoming flowers, and in the squeals of small children.

I know of no better way to acknowledge God than to sit still and be quiet. We can prepare to enter this divine communion through the vocalization of words, scriptures, or songs, but we must remember that these are only preparations for a deeper communion with the Absolute. Recognizing our oneness with the Source of all life, and being aware of and receptive to the grace that is flowing to us in the stillness of being, is the heart of authentic prayer. And when we go into prayer, we go for only one reason: to seek God and have communion with God. We do not go to seek counsel, to ask guidance, or to seek healing, prosperity, or a job. We do not attempt to get God to do something for us, to triumph over the "evil" we perceive is happening in our lives.

If you go to God just to get God to fix something that is

"going wrong" in your life, you're missing the point and power of prayer. God is not in the employment, real estate, medical, or any other service-oriented business. God is in the business of helping us recognize His presence and His power and His goodness in us. God's life in us is what He wants to radiate outward to others. Investing time with God will enable you to set your mind like a trap in order to catch the wisdom and thoughts of God. And of course, if you follow the guidance you receive, everything you need will be added.

If you learn to acknowledge God by being aware of His presence continually in the ways we will discuss in this chapter, your spiritual digestive system will automatically receive the food of God's light-energy and distribute it where it ought to go in your life. The more you concentrate consciously on the presence of God within you, the more your total being begins to digest that light-energy until all of your pores and cells are radiating the energy of God.

The most important thing to expect in prayer is contact with God. That is why meditation is so powerful. Unless we are quiet, how can we open our mind to set a trap to catch the thoughts of God? A hunter has to lie in wait, breathing quietly but in a state of complete alertness, if he wants to catch his prey. The mind in its normal state is never still enough to catch the thoughts of God. We prosper and live an abundant life by experiencing God as God reveals Himself. Many of these revelations can be found in the "I AMs" that Jesus pronounced. Jesus never said that the human person known as Jesus of Nazareth was the "resurrection and the life." The Gospel says that God raised Jesus from the dead; it doesn't say a thing about Jesus raising himself.

So then, who raised Jesus? The eternal "I AM." The name "Yeshua" means "I AM saves." Jesus was referring to the in-dwelling Spirit of "I AM" as "the resurrection and the life." When you begin to acknowledge God as the eternal, ever-present "I AM," then your fears will begin to diminish. At that point you can say with the psalmist, in effect, "What is there to fear?"

When we enter into prayer, we are recipients of the divine electricity of the Holy Spirit flowing to us upon request. When I pray for people, I simply welcome the Holy Spirit into the situation by saying, "Come, Holy Spirit." The moment I make the request for that divine electrical presence to occur, I know it's here. This does not imply that I am better than anyone else. I'm simply attempting to demonstrate to others that they may release this divine energy into their own lives as well as into the lives of others. You do not have to beg or plead for the Holy Spirit to come.

The awareness that light-energy is coming to you in this time of communion with God is the answer to your prayer. Results will follow in one form or another. People want the answer to their prayers to be in words. They want direct guidance from someone or a promise that tomorrow is going to be all right. Yet the instant our thoughts are focused on God, the eternal I AM, that I AM–ness is activated in our lives. The paradox is that from that point on, we have no need for words or thoughts.

To be fully receptive to God's intentions in the way I am describing, perhaps we need to rekindle our faith in miracles and rediscover the mystical in the everyday. In his book *Riding with the Lion: In Search of Mystical Christianity*, Greek Orthodox author Kyriacos Markides writes that one of the problems with Christianity as represented by the organized churches of the various denominations is that "they have become so secularized that they have banished that which is at the core of all religion—the reality of miracles, of mystery and faith." Christianity was established on miracles, on spiritual phenomena. Yet today we see at one extreme a kind of intellectual religion and at the other, an entertainment religion; neither of these represents the authentic path of Jesus the man or Jesus the Christ. Catholicism, Orthodoxy, and many Protestant sects have, generally speaking, fallen into rigid intellectual ritualism and alienated the hearts of their followers. Meanwhile, the Pentecostal and Evangelical churches have become extremely radical in their emotionalism and entertainment approach to Christianity. Some perpetuate the message of prosperity without the message of sacrifice, and have lost their roots. Saint Paul said, "Let your roots go down deep into God's love."

Spirituality can, however, embrace the miraculous and also avoid attachment to material prosperity and health as ends in themselves. When you pray, be detached from the outcome. Christ's saying "Blessed are the poor in spirit" has been misinterpreted as "Blessed are the poor." In monastic Christianity, poverty didn't mean being impoverished, it meant being detached.

One of the great liberating developments in modern Western spirituality has been an increasing openness to other, especially Eastern, traditions. Many Westerners have been attracted to the various Indian, Chinese, and Japanese traditions almost certainly by their techniques of knowing God directly and intimately through meditation, yoga, and chanting. These practices have provided a kind of antidote or balance to the intellectualized approach of most Western religions. Now it is time to realize that our Western traditions are rich in spiritual practices of their own, methods that have long been buried within the mystical practices that haven't been made accessible to most Christians, Jews, or Muslims by their religious institutions. Some of the Christian methods are remarkably simple and often quite similar to the devotional practices of early Christian laypeople, whose role has often been downplayed or denigrated by church hierarchies.

As a child growing up in a Catholic household, for instance, I was taught to offer prayers to God called "ejaculations"—short phrases that even then I recognized as energizing. In the wake of the reforms of Vatican II, grassroots mystical practices such as this have lost favor, but I would encourage you to reclaim them and reshape them as your own. For example, when sad, lonely, or depressed, I would become still and repeat ejaculations like "My Jesus, mercy," "My God and my All," or "Almighty God, be with me." Almost instantly these miniature prayers released spiritual overtones that resonated within my being, sending tiny vibrations of energy up and down my spine. The sadness, loneliness, or depression generally lifted.

I urge you to do the same when your energy level seems to be depleted. Better yet, do it while you are at a high energy level—why wait? Sit down quietly and take your spiritual medication by repeating a short prayer that is deeply significant to you, such as "The Lord is my Shepherd" or "Sacred Heart of Jesus." Breathe deeply and be aware of your breath as you are aware of the words you are saying. Be aware, too, of the feelings generated in your body and the atmosphere around you. Do this for five to ten minutes. Then return to your usual activities until you feel led to practice this form of prayer again. As a priest, you are privileged to be one with God and keep that connection. You can experience God's presence continually with you and within you. Remember that your calling as a priest is from God, not from some institution claiming to speak for God. You personally have been invited to an intimate relationship with the Almighty. Through this relationship, you have been graced with the energy of ordination and another opportunity to achieve wholeness.

One of Mahatma Gandhi's favorite methods of prayer was what he called "the repetition of Ramanama," or praying by repeating the name of God (the technique is also known by the Sanskrit term *japa* or *japanama*). Whenever Gandhi was afflicted with dysentery, he would forgo medication. Instead he would tell his aides to leave him alone for a time, during which he would repeat the name of Rama and from which he would emerge in good health. He called this practice of Ramanama "the poor man's medicine." That is also the idea behind the Buddhist *nembutsu* prayer developed in twelfth-century Japan, which required only the repetition of the phrase *"Namu Amida Butsu,"* or "Veneration to Amida Buddha." Likewise in the Russian Orthodox "Jesus Prayer," developed from the prayers of the Desert Fathers of the third and fourth centuries, you repeat, "Lord Jesus Christ, Son of the living God, have mercy on me, a sinner" (or a shorter variation) until it goes from the head to the heart.

When you pronounce a name with love, any name, you make a connection with it. I can look at a picture of my mother, who died a few years ago, and call upon her name and feel an immediate connection. Now you might say that's just memory or affection, but I would disagree. In the act of love, we call our beloved's name and it seems to release an energy in our beloved as it does in us. Take that concept to a higher frequency by calling on the name of God and you begin to see the power that simple prayer can unleash.

Most of the wisdom traditions are aware of this. In the Muslim tradition, for instance, especially among Sufis, the faithful chant what are known as the Ninety-nine Beautiful Names of Allah, which are actually various attributes or identities of God, such as *Raheem* ("Beneficent"), *Rahman* ("Merciful"), or *Nur* ("Light"). These names can be chanted under one's breath during the activities of the day, in brief bursts of prayer, or in sessions known as *zhikrs* that can go on for hours at a time. This is the same principle behind the Roman Catholic and Orthodox litanies of the Holy Name of Jesus or of the Blessed Mother, as you can see from the following lines I've selected from each of those two popular litanies. (Traditionally, the priest says these invocations and after each one the faithful repeat, "Pray for us.")

Jesus, splendor of the Creator,
Jesus, brightness of eternal light,
Jesus, king of glory,
Jesus, lover of the human family,
Jesus, unbounded goodness.

LITANY OF THE HOLY NAME

Virgin, powerful in the sight of God,
Mirror of holiness,
Seat of wisdom,
Shrine of the spirit,
Mystical rose,
Tower of ivory,
House of gold,
Ark of the Covenant,
Health of the sick.

LITANY OF OUR LADY

In a real sense, this kind of practice is not so different from my understanding of the Rosary. I always carry one of my rosaries with me on which to pray. I do not always pray on it in the usual way. I don't strive to complete five decades in one sitting but to enter into a state during which, after just three Hail Marys, I can achieve a kind of bliss uncluttered by words or thoughts. Or I may say on each bead, "Lord, mercy. Lord, mercy. Lord, mercy." Hindus and Buddhists have long used some form of prayer beads, and the Christian and Muslim rosaries are doubtless descended from theirs. Some cultures call them "worry beads," because as the faithful finger them, their attention goes to God and that alleviates their worry. But using the beads also facilitates doing what Saint Paul advises, and that is to pray without ceasing. As Paramahansa Yogananda wrote in his beautiful poem "God! God! God!":

No matter where I go, the spotlight of my mind
Ever keeps turning on Thee;
And in the battle din of activity my silent war-cry is ever:
God! God! God!

. . . .

In waking, eating, working, dreaming, sleeping,
Serving, meditating, chanting, divinely loving,
My soul constantly hums, unheard by any:
God! God! God!

Most mornings, I spend two to three hours in prayer. Although that may be somewhat more than the average person devotes to daily prayer and meditation, and may even appear extreme, it's not a great deal of time compared to the life of many monastics and mystics. Yet I never do the same thing every day. Some days I may come downstairs and be guided to pray the Rosary. Other times I may take up the beads and say an affirmation on each bead instead of a Hail Mary. Or I might be guided to choose a spiritual book and read from it. Every one of these activities brings me almost instantly into a connection I so enjoy that I don't want to come out of it in less than two or three hours.

For those who haven't spent years developing a prayer life, however, the sources of prayer may not come so easily. I can recommend several simple approaches. One I especially like is to take a different attribute of God and devote a week to meditating on it. If a long meditation is impractical because of your schedule or because you haven't developed the endurance yet, you can take an attribute of God and bring it into your consciousness at ten or twenty different times during the course of a day. Each time might last only one minute, but the residual effect is to call your attention continually back to God.

In the beginning, it may be difficult to remember to do this ten or twenty times a day, simply because we become so absorbed in work or play or troubles. But the trick is to remember God in the midst of these. Try leaving little cards or Post-it notes of a certain color in various places around the house—on the refrigerator, the toilet, the bathroom mirror, in your car, or on the job, depending on where you spend the most time (for me, that would probably be the refrigerator). Once you get into the habit of remembering God in these small moments and everyday activities, you may not need to keep the notes up. Eventually the intention will become strong enough for you to keep recalling God throughout the day. If you have a digital wristwatch with an hourly chime feature, set it to chime on the hour and each time you hear the chime, take the next minute to focus on the relevant attribute of God.

MEDITATIONS ON THE ATTRIBUTES OF GOD

Here is a sample list of seven attributes that you can use:

Week 1: Mercy

Week 2: Kindness

Week 3: Pure light

Week 4: Omnipotence

Week 5: Omniscience

Week 6: Omnipresence

Week 7: Health

Take a few deep breaths to relax your body and calm your mind. If any negative thoughts come to you, let them pass by. (Just say to them, "Thank you for sharing," and let them go!) Take into your consciousness, first, the attribute of Mercy. Say the word reverently two or three times aloud, if you are in a situation that allows this. If you are at work or among people, you may just think the word or say it silently. Then relax and allow the Holy Spirit to paint the picture of God as Mercy upon the canvas of your mind. If you are a Buddhist, the Spirit may paint a picture of merciful actions of the Buddha. Depending on your tradition or what appeals to you, you may see a saintly human being, whether it's Ramana Maharshi, Mother Teresa, Mansur al-Hallaj, Rabbi Hillel, Confucius, or Lao-tzu. Stay with that awhile.

Don't try to visualize. In visualization, we strive to create a picture ourselves. There's nothing wrong with that, but that is different from arriving at the point where God paints the picture. The mystics called this contemplation. In visualization, we do the work; in contemplation, God does the work.

In some ways it's easier to relegate half an hour in the morning and half an hour at night to prayer or meditation, but that leaves a large gap of time during the day in which you are not reminding yourself of God. In practicing energetic and healing prayer, however, the whole idea is to bring His presence constantly into remembrance. Try saying the prayer ejaculations I mentioned throughout the day in place of remembering the attributes of God. But don't just say the ejaculations; allow yourself a minute to watch what starts coming up for you when you suddenly turn your focus to God. Bring your awareness to the practice and discipline of prayer. That way, when any fears and tribulations come on you down the road, you can continue to remind yourself of the presence of God and draw on the strength and energy that emanate from that awareness.

According to Muslim tradition, one night while the Prophet Muhammad slept he was taken on a night journey to the Temple in Jerusalem. There he prayed with Abraham, Moses, and Jesus before ascending a celestial ladder of seven planes of being to the seventh heaven and beyond, where he communed with the formless God and was dazzled by the beatific vision. Allah commanded Muhammad to have his people vow to pray fifty times a day. Moses, stationed a level or two below, approached the Prophet as he descended and when he heard of the Lord's command, urged him to go back and ask for a more realistic vow. Muhammad returned, and God agreed to reduce the number of prayer breaks to forty. This still sounded excessive to Moses, who, in the venerable Semitic tradition reaching back to Abraham of haggling with God for the sake of humanity, insisted that Muhammad bargain for fewer prayers. After a series of intercessions, God finally reduced the number of daily prayers to five. Although Moses advised Muhammad to negotiate a still better deal, Muhammad was loath to ask again, and Muslim law was set. The idea of praying at distinct times during the day was already part of the Christian mystical tradition that is still reflected in the saying of the Daily Office, the system of seven daytime hours and one night office observed by priests and monks of the Catholic and Eastern Orthodox traditions. The great innovation of Muhammad in the seventh century, however, was to bring this mystical practice into the daily lives of *all* the faithful.

In thirteenth-century Italy, the Catholic Church initiated the practice of saying the Angelus at morning, noon, and evening hours, when a set of three Hail Marys and other prayers was signaled for all to hear by the ringing of the church bells. This devotional practice was immortalized by Jean François Millet's famous painting depicting a peasant couple who have stopped their toil in the fields to pray with heads bowed. (In my own community of Peru, Illinois, only the local Polish church of Saint Valentine's maintains the tradition of ringing the Angelus bells.) In the Jewish tradition, the faithful are expected to recite the *Sh'ma* four times a day—twice during morning prayers, once during the evening service, and again at home just before bedtime. The *Sh'ma,* a single verse from Deuteronomy (6:4)—"Hear, O Israel, the Lord is Our God, the Lord is One," or in Hebrew, *"Sh'ma Yisra'el, Adonai Elo-heinu, Adonai Ehad"*—probably comes the closest of all Jewish prayers to encapsulating the essence of Jewish belief.

As modern mystics, we are free to borrow from all these traditions and to shape them in our own way just as the mystics of the various traditions themselves have done. The Sufis, who delved the mystical depths of Islam, for instance, elaborated on the five-times-daily prayers by developing ways of keeping the names of Allah on their breath all day long. In the beginning, the most important thing is the intention of praying continually. Say to yourself, "I intend to do this ten times today." It may seem superficial at first, but at some point it will become a part of you, like eating breakfast, going for your daily walk, or brushing your teeth.

You can find plenty of reminders if you set your mind to it. I keep a chaplet rosary (a little less than half the length of a standard rosary) on my desk during the day, and that reminds me to stop at different times. I may not pray all twenty-five beads when I pick up the chaplet, but it is a good reminder of my intention to stop ten times and bring some sacred word or phrase into my consciousness. I have a lot of sacred statues and icons around my house, but they don't work as well as the beads do to remind me—maybe because I associate the beads with prayer tools. I also carry beads in my pocket as a reminder when I'm out walking or traveling by train or plane.

Some of you may have unpleasant associations with objects like rosaries because of your religious upbringing. The Star of David or the Miraculous Medal may remind you of the pious kids in your Hebrew or Catholic parochial school or, conversely, of the tough kids who wore them as jewelry or talismans with no special spiritual significance. You can reclaim these objects for yourself and give them new meaning. For instance, if you are at your desk and you have a medal around your neck that you consider to be a spiritual tool, you can put your finger on it to remind you to open the heart chakra. As Padre Pio once said, "If prayer does not lead to love, it is not prayer." If you have an image of the Sacred Heart in your mind and this represents God's unconditional love for you, you can tap the medal or your own heart. At first, because you have not been taught to be aware of this, you may not feel anything, but eventually you may begin to feel tingling vibrations moving through your body.

These are just some of the tools I use to draw my mind back to the Parent of all life, or what George Fowler calls the "Source Being." Many people even have a problem with the name "God" itself because of the way they were raised, so a phrase like Source Being may be more acceptable to them. Familiarize yourself with the name of God in other traditions, whether it's Rama or Rahman, and if you prefer, use those instead of the standard Christian or Jewish names. In the end, the name you have for God is considerably less important than the state of consciousness you enter into when you repeat it.

Healing Prayers, Meditations, and Sacred Verses for Daily Use

The daily process I use to anchor myself in the presence of God is a simple one that can easily be divided into four steps. The overall process entails choosing a scriptural passage or reading a book until a sentence inspires or moves you in some way, then bringing that sentence into your consciousness and repeating it until the very words themselves dissolve into nothing. That may last only a split second for the beginner, but in that moment you have entered the halls of contemplation where God reveals Himself. Here now are the four steps in detail. Please read them all through before beginning the exercise.

Step 1. Take spiritual truth into your consciousness. I use a scripture passage or a sacred writing, such as the words of people I consider to be saints or mystics—those who have experienced God in such a way as to be able to share the truth of what they've learned with others. They would be able to take that truth into their spirit and allow the Spirit of God to make it grow within them, enabling God's energy to radiate outward so others can feel the power of the words.

Step 2. Practice centering upon that truth in a word or phrase until you enter a state of meditation. I call this stage guided imaging led by the Spirit of God. Focus every part of your being on the word or phrase you have selected so as to let the Holy Spirit embrace it and make it real for you. You then enter into a state of meditation through guided imagery that is led by God's Holy Spirit. This is not an attempt to make things happen on a mental level.

Step 3. As God's Spirit leads you through this sacred imagery, begin to feel His presence. You will enter into a state of contemplation where you rest in the presence of God, experiencing the healing light, love, and presence, but you use no words or thoughts. If any thoughts come to your mind during the time, let them pass through. Do not struggle with the thoughts or judge yourself for having them. As you return again to the words upon which you are focusing, you will begin to know that the word is not the important thing. The important thing is to be aware of the stillness in the centering process, for in that stillness you will experience the eternal "I

AM." In this state of contemplation, you are resting in the presence of "I AM" and you are simply learning to receive.

Step 4. Conclude with acts of gratitude and thanks, which primarily consist not only of words but also of bringing God's love to others. There is nothing wrong with singing to God, praising and worshiping God, or praying the Psalms to God. The greatest act of gratitude to God for His presence in your life, however, is to go out into the world and show that presence in love available to whoever will need to be in your presence. You don't have to search for them; God will bring them to you.

Prior to Step 1, read a passage of sacred writing. As an example, I will take a New Testament reading on the Transfiguration, centering on the phrase "God is light." Then I will quietly allow the Holy Spirit to reveal to me exactly what that means.

> After six days, Jesus took Peter, John, and James with Him and went up a high mountain where they were all alone. There Jesus was transfigured before them. His clothes became dazzling white, whiter than any bleached garment. There appeared before them Elijah and Moses, who were talking with Jesus. Peter said to Jesus, "Teacher, it is good for us to be here. . . ." Then a cloud appeared and enveloped them. And a voice came from the cloud. "This is my Son whom I love dearly; listen to Him."

I will now take the phrase "God is light" into my consciousness and condense it into one word for my meditative purpose: "light." Having done my part by allowing the Holy Spirit to take over and guide me to the fuller awareness of God's presence as "light," I can relax. In the deep silence of contemplation, we touch the hem of the Christ's garment, allowing God to reveal Himself as love, mercy, compassion, forgiveness, tenderness, and light.

As you enter into this exercise, you may want to have a sacred object upon which you can focus, depending on your religious background and what is comfortable for you. This object can be a picture of Jesus, a Miraculous Medal or crucifix, an image of the Buddha or Shiva or Lao-tzu, the Tetragrammaton or Kabbalistic Tree of Life, or a painting that touches you deeply. You may want to play music you consider sacred. You may also wish to light a perfumed candle. There is no magic in any of these items. They are reminders of our connection with God through which we receive spiritual energy. Remind yourself that whatever tools you use are to help you with this holy moment of encounter. Tools such as I have mentioned help me to prepare for the holy moment of my encounter with God daily. I know they will do the same for you.

This exercise ought to be performed fifteen minutes upon awakening and fifteen minutes prior to sleep. You should also consider adding brief prayer breaks of one or two minutes at least ten times a day, to reconnect consciously with the Presence of God. The two exercises that follow can be used throughout the day in ways that I have described in this chapter. You may want to try each one for a week or two to discover which method works best for you.

EXERCISE FOR BATHING IN LIGHT-ENERGY

What do I mean when I say that you must allow your mind and your heart to be bathed by the light-energy, the Spirit of God? Essentially you are to receive and release thoughts of love, peace, forgiveness, and mercy. Here is a little exercise for you to do in the coming week. During your time of devotion, take into your hands some prayer beads—and it doesn't matter if they are Hindu, Buddhist, Catholic, or Sufi rosary beads—and with each bead, say, "God is the one power." Keep repeating that sentence until you get to the point where you recognize that from this one power flows all the goodness of God. If you don't need such beads to help you focus, then simply repeat the words. Release light thoughts, which contain the rhythmic, vibrational energy of God's love. Some of these light thoughts are added in the Appendixes of this book in the form of words contained in various sacred writings as well as personal prayers.

The following week, rather than doing this exercise during your regular devotional time, do something else during that time but carry your beads with you in your pocket or purse. Whenever you have free time—whether you're walking down the street, riding a bus or subway, standing on line in the bank or supermarket—finger your beads and repeat, "God is the one power" on each bead. You don't have to carry your beads publicly; you can leave them in your pocket and say the prayer silently. The important thing is to find new ways and places to work the repeated prayer into your daily routine.

MOMENTARY PRAYER EXERCISE

Here is a brief spiritual exercise that you can say at any time during the day when you have a few minutes to sit in a quiet spot. Although it is effective when done by yourself, you can also do this exercise with a group of people.

Begin by closing your eyes and taking three deep breaths. Then seek the guidance of that element of God called the Holy

Spirit, saying, "Do with me what you will. Show me how I can better serve my brothers and sisters."

Make this prayer an expression of your desire to grow spiritually and not be afraid of God. If you are doing this as a group exercise, take the hand of the person next to you. If not, place your hands in your lap, one on top of the other, palms facing upward. Then say to yourself, "Come, Spirit of God. Reveal your presence. Come, Spirit of the living God. I am receptive. I welcome you."

You may experience phenomena such as heat, cooling, or tingling sensations, or you may begin to vibrate or to feel a numbness in your body. All sorts of phenomena may happen when you open yourself to God. Just let them be.

Then ask yourself this closing question: "May I be of assistance to God as a channel through which the Spirit of Life, the energy of God, can be given expression?"

Now thank God for your life exactly as it is, not as you would like it to be. Then open your eyes and take several more deep breaths before going on with your daily life.

FOUR

THE LORD'S PRAYER: A NEW PERSPECTIVE

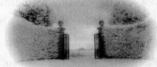

In all the religions of humankind, the sacred teachings have always been written down in the language of the founder.

◆

NEIL DOUGLAS-KLOTZ, *PRAYERS OF THE COSMOS*

Although the New Testament was written in Greek and the Old Testament in Hebrew, Jesus spoke Aramaic, the lingua franca of the region, when he preached to the people of Judea. Greek was spoken mainly by the educated classes, and Hebrew had long since become a largely sacred language reserved for use by the Temple priests. (It would not become a living language again until the twentieth century, shortly before the establishment of the State of Israel.) Aramaic, an ancient tongue that has linguistic links to both Hebrew and Arabic, is considered by many scholars to be older than either of those languages. When the Aramaic words of Jesus were first translated into the Greek of the Gospels, much of their original intent was obscured because of the great difference between the two tongues. Subsequent retranslation into Latin, Old English, and modern English has only worsened those initial distortions, and has helped embed them in our consciousness.

We can recapture the original meaning of the teachings of Jesus, however, by looking at the language in which Jesus thought and taught to see what the words can tell us about his true intentions. Biblical scholars generally agree that the Gospels were not written down in the Greek on which all current translations are based until at least forty years after Christ's crucifixion. Some of these scholars conjecture that the Gospel accounts, which were not written by eyewitnesses bearing the names of the four Evangelists, may have been based on an Aramaic original of which no copy has yet been found.

Although we do not have that original Aramaic manuscript, we do have something known as the Peshitta Version of the Syriac Aramaic manuscript of the Gospels, which some Eastern Christian scholars believe dates from the second century A.D. Although that would make it even further removed from the time of Jesus than the Gospels, it has the advantage of having been written in the language Jesus spoke, and so probably reflects a more faithful version of his teachings. The discussion that follows is derived from various scholarly readings of the Peshitta, and is largely based on the work of George M. Lamsa, Rocco A. Errico, and Neil Douglas-Klotz, among others. My revision of the Lord's Prayer is a compilation of these scholars' works expanded by my own understanding of this prayer as I have used it in my spiritual healing work.

Most readers know the Lord's Prayer as it is said today in almost all the world's English-speaking Christian churches:

> Our Father, who art in heaven, hallowed be thy name.
> Thy kingdom come, thy will be done on earth, as it is in
> heaven. Give us this day our daily bread, and forgive us
> our trespasses as we forgive those who trespass against
> us. Lead us not into temptation, but deliver us from evil.

The Protestant version concludes,

> For thine is the kingdom, and the power, and the glory,
> for ever and ever. Amen.

In the Aramaic spoken by Jesus, however, the Lord's Prayer would read much more like this:

> Our Father, who is everywhere in the universe, your
> name is sacred. Your kingdom is come among us, your

will is throughout the earth as it is throughout the universe. You give us our needful bread from day to day and you forgive us our offenses even as we forgive our offenders. You do not let us enter into materialism, but you separate us from error. For yours is the kingdom, and the power, and the song, from ages to ages. Sealed in faithfulness.

At first blush, the two versions may seem to differ only superficially in style and syntax. Yet what is the first thing you notice about the second version as opposed to the Our Father that you have always known? Every statement of Jesus in the Aramaic was an affirmation or a declaration of truth, whereas the Our Father as it has been translated from the Greek culminates in a long string of petitions. When Jesus taught the people to pray (probably over a period of days, later collated by his disciples into a single prayer), he was saying to the people, in essence, This is what you can expect from God. It was the spiritual equivalent of "We hold these truths to be self-evident." You need not ask for what is already accomplished in the universe, Jesus was saying. All you need to know is how to accept it. If you doubt that was his perspective, take a look at the verses just preceding the Lord's Prayer in the Gospel of Matthew (6:7–8). After telling his followers not to "heap up empty phrases as the Gentiles do" (and as most of us, sadly, have been taught to do), he adds, "Do not be like them, for your Father knows what you need before you ask him." If God already knows what we need, why ask at all? Better to affirm.

This difference in syntax has great significance for how we understand the message of Jesus. He is telling us, in effect, that what keeps us healthy is the awareness that we don't have to ask for health. Sickness and poverty are not judgments from God or the karmic residue of some evil we committed in a past life. They may, of course, be largely the result of unhealthful living habits or bad financial planning, but those can be corrected. If you are sickly or impoverished, declare that God wants to give you your daily bread and that God's will is to separate you from all error that occurs in your thinking. This clearly reflects a loving and compassionate God, far removed from the blood-and-thunder of the Old Testament God. How did Jesus exemplify this change in conceptualizing our Divine Parent?

When you go to the Father, Jesus said, the first thing you need to understand is that your Father is a Daddy. The Aramaic word Jesus used is *Abba* or *Abwoon,* which is closer to "Papa" or "Daddy" than to the more formal "Father." Rocco Errico points out that when people prayed in those days, they were likely to say, "Oh, Father Abraham," or "Oh, Father Jacob," calling on the patriarchs to mediate with God in their behalf. Jesus is telling us that we can go directly to the Father and address Him as intimately as a child approaching his Dad, because he is not some distant, fearful figure but a Being of light and love. Jesus is saying that God is concerned about everything that concerns you, and if your Daddy loves you unconditionally, there is nothing you need ask that he has not already supplied. All you need do is declare to yourself that this is the truth. You need not ask for anything, because if you have to ask for it, you are living an error. Our role as children of God is to accept into our life that this is what God wants to do for us.

To understand more fully the concept of prayer as medication for the spirit, soul, and body, we have to understand how Jesus saw the Father, how he saw the world and the people around him. And to understand his world, we have to return for a moment to the language of his day. The two most ancient sacred languages we know of are Sanskrit and Aramaic. In Sanskrit, the word for prayer is *pal al. Pal al* can best be translated "seeing oneself as wondrously made." If you are going to communicate with God, then you must see yourself as wondrously made, which is to say, made in the image of God as Spirit. The essence of your being is the light of God, the energy of God, the Spirit of God. All of this represented a new concept for the people of Jesus' time, who had forgotten that God was a Daddy. They still saw God as a punitive Being ready to punish them for their transgressions—the way many fundamentalists see God today.

Since, as noted earlier, the sense of the Aramaic word for "prayer" is "to set a trap," when you enter into the presence of God to communicate with Him, you focus your attention as if you were a hunter waiting patiently to catch the thoughts of God. The whole idea of prayer, then, isn't so much about talking to God as it is about listening to God. To pray means to tune in, on a spiritual wavelength, to the consciousness of God. The energy of God, as I've also noted, is always being broadcast. God never says, "Today I'm turning off my broadcasting system. I'm not going to pour out any more love because I'm tired." He is always broadcasting love, compassion, and forgiveness, and on that frequency flows the energy to heal, restore, make whole, and revive. In authentic prayer, we prepare our hearts and minds to receive God's energy by attuning ourselves to Him.

The origins of the English word "God" are somewhat obscure. It's tempting to say it is cognate with the German *gut,* meaning "good," but the original derivation may reach back through Anglo-Saxon and Old German to the past participle of a Sanskrit word meaning "he calls upon (a god)" or "conjures up," suggesting a more ancient, magical conception. The Aramaic word for what would be translated as God is *Alaha,* from which were derived the Arabic *Allah* and the Hebrew *Elohim. Alaha* means "essence" or "substance of all being." When the Jews of Jesus' time and place used the Aramaic word for God, they were denoting the substance out of which everything else is created. *Alaha,* then, would signify to Aramaic-speaking people "breath" or "life force." When they prayed to God, they were communicating with the Life Force of all creation. To them, prayer was not the words you say to God, but rather your life with God. When Aramaic-speaking people made a connection with the Creator, it was as humans connecting with the Divine in the awareness that every breath is an inhalation of the divine presence.

From the foregoing, it should be clear that we are talking about different conceptions of God existing side by side in the Judea of Jesus' day. As with most of the world's religions, the institutional or intellectual understanding of God purveyed by the religious leaders of the day was probably at odds with the ancient mystical tradition. In India, for instance, we know that the formulaic, priest-ridden Vedic religion brought to the Indus Valley by the invading Aryans was integrated over time with the preexisting yogic mysticism of the indigenous peoples. What we today call Hinduism can refer to either or both of these traditions. Likewise in the Aramaic-speaking countryside where Jesus lived and taught, conceptions of God must have varied enormously. In *Prayers of the Cosmos,* Neil Douglas-Klotz writes,

> Native peoples of the Middle East also had a rich language, culture, and spirituality for thousands of years before Jesus. His inspired use of many older sacred phrases, reaching back even before the Hebrew tradition, shows that a native mystical tradition did survive, probably in hiding or in the desert, both before and throughout the rise of orthodox Judaism, Christianity, and Islam. Some schools of Sufism claim to be among the inheritors of this native Middle Eastern tradition, which precedes even the Egyptian mystery schools.

In that time and place, the threatening image of a distant, unapproachable God whose name one dared not utter existed alongside an understanding of God as the very breath of life. This more immediate, loving God was probably known to a handful of mystics and desert dwellers and to some extent to communities like the Essenes, but was not being widely broadcast before Jesus arrived. The great gift he bestowed on the world was to make the intimate knowledge of God as loving Parent available to the masses. No wonder elements of the Jewish religious establishment and the Roman colonial occupying forces were equally appalled at this man who offered one of the earliest manifestations of Power to the People!

The Aramaic understanding of God as the divine breath that created all the universe and that has the power to restore and heal can also permeate our spiritual life today. Every time you inhale with that awareness, you begin to believe in the possibility that the energy of God enters into you with every breath. Every time you exhale, all of the spiritual toxic waste goes back out into the universe where the light, love, and heat of God's Spirit is present and dissolves it.

As you begin to pray with this awareness, you ought to start seeing a change, not simply in your inner being but also in your physical body. Our bodies are regularly and completely reconstituted with new cells. At least once every three years we receive what amounts to a new body—and even more frequently for the skin and certain tissues and organs. Yet if every cell is being transformed, why does the body still maintain its cancer, its diabetes, its HIV-positive status? Perhaps change on a cellular level is dependent on our belief system and filters the energy of God through it. The scriptures constantly remind us to change our thinking, to be transformed by renewing our thought patterns. Put on the mind that was in Christ Jesus, Paul tells us. In teaching the Lord's Prayer, Jesus was demonstrating to his followers how to change their thinking, how to change the mind to receive everything God wants to give us.

We are living in a spiritual universe because we are not really this matter that we seem to be. Our body is just the form that the energy is taking at this point. The Indian mystic Ramana Maharshi constantly reminded his followers to ask themselves, Who am I? If I am not this mind and I am not this body, who am I? He would often ask them this question until they ran out of answers and were finally stunned into silence. In one sense the answer is simple: We are spirit. But since there is no simple definition or explanation of spirit, maybe silence is the best answer after all.

If spirit cannot be explained, at least we can acknowledge that it exists and is indestructible. The mind and body will decay and become one with the earth again, but spiritual energy cannot die. The spiritual universe we live in is alive, dynamic, filled with light and energy. In such a universe, God is understood intuitively, which is the true nature of intelligence as God created us.

We are often amazed when someone appears to be able to read minds. And yet if we accept the nature of the universe as essentially spiritual, and if one can have a strong connection with God and by extension with every living creation of God, then the act of intuiting another's thoughts becomes less mystifying. Once again, that is precisely what Jesus meant when he said that if you have faith, nothing is impossible. Some of us are attuned to our intuition and we receive our hunches loud and clear. If you are so attuned, when you meet certain people you may intuit that they are not good to relate to. It isn't that you don't like their hairdo or the way they talk, or that you think you're "above" them; it's that you are receiving, on a gut or energetic level, exactly what they are feeling about you.

Once you begin to open yourself to such feelings and allow yourself to become aware of them, you are beginning to live by the

Spirit. You may even be on the path to becoming clairvoyant, clairaudient, or prophetic, or to becoming a healer, simply because you understand on the heart level.

I'm not out to demean logic or rational thought. In some ways, we use genuine logic far too little at times, and are ruled by emotions and impulses that are insufficiently understood or controlled. All I'm saying is that logic and reason are not who we are. When Jesus spoke to people, he communicated on the level of who they really were—Spirit to spirit.

As Jesus' words were translated from the Aramaic, too much was unfortunately lost, and our spirit can easily miss the Spirit he was trying to communicate. In the case of the Lord's Prayer, as I've noted, a whole series of positive affirmations turned into a series of petitions to God. But Jesus' meaning was subtly distorted in other ways as well. For instance, Jesus told his disciples to pray and to heal in his name. Over the ensuing two thousand years, that request has degenerated into using the name of Jesus like a rabbit's foot. Some believe that if you tack that phrase onto any prayer or request for healing, it will carry greater weight with the Father. We often hear television healers, for instance, pray for a healing "In Jesus' name. Amen!" That wasn't what Jesus meant at all when he told his followers to pray in his name. If I said in Aramaic to do something "in my name," the meaning would be to do it "as I would do it."

In this case, if I tell you to pray in the name of Jesus, then you and I must have the same understanding of the attributes and essence of God's nature that Jesus had. We have to share the same concept of creation and our oneness with it that Jesus had. And we have to have the same basic understanding that the primal energy of the universe is the word of God spoken.

Whenever Jesus approached the Father, he knew exactly Whom he was approaching. Many of us don't. He knew exactly what the will of the Father was. Most of us don't. In fact, many of us add to our prayers the condition "If it be Thy will." At first, this may sound like a selfless and humble phrase, as when Muslims interject the Arabic qualifier *"Insh'allah,"* or "God willing." And yet if you understand the personality of God as Daddy, then you know that the will of God is His unconditional desire to grant gifts and the abundant life and sense of fulfillment to His children.

The Aramaic word *besheme,* which has been translated in the New Testament as "in my name," actually means "according to my approach or my way of doing things." Jesus meant, "When you pray, pray in this manner, with this approach. State from the beginning, Our Daddy who is everywhere present." The message is clear: When you approach God, don't stand in a corner begging and pleading. Enter in all humility but enter with your head high into the presence of your Daddy who is everywhere. There is no place in the universe where an individual can be that God is not.

One of the Psalms says, "Even if my soul go down into Sheol [the Hebrew equivalent of hell, without the hellfire], You are there." God is approachable and available to everyone. He is not just the Father of Christians but also of Hindus and Buddhists and atheists. God is approachable and available to everyone. If God is available to everyone and he is everyone's Daddy, then there is no need for a mediator. As we begin to pray, we tune ourselves in to the fact that we are already one with the Goodness of the universe.

Let's examine the Lord's Prayer one phrase at a time and see if we can begin to understand what Jesus was actually saying, as opposed to the words his translators have put into his mouth.

The opening phrase, "Our Father who art in heaven," could more accurately be rendered "Our Father (or Daddy) who is everywhere in the universe" or "Our Universal Father." Rocco Errico makes note of the fact that the word "God" appears nowhere in this prayer. And since we tend, after years of religious training, to think of "heaven" as a distant realm up above the sky, it may be more constructive to realize that the Divine Parent exists everywhere in the universe, above and below, around and within. As Jesus said in the Gnostic Gospel of Thomas, "Lift a stone and you will find me; cleave the wood and I am there."

"Hallowed be thy name" in the original Aramaic would be better translated as "Your name is sacred." In other words, "Your name, God, is set aside for a specific purpose and is not to be used for any other reason." That is why Jesus told the people not to take oaths as was the custom of the time. When a merchant sold goods in the marketplace, he might swear, "By God, my weights are correct!" Here we see the relationship of the Old Testament commandment not to take the name of the Lord your God in vain spelled out more precisely. If the name of God has power and a purpose, which is to release the energy of all goodness, we must not take it in vain or use it in an empty way because this will only dissipate its power.

"Your kingdom is come" literally means that God's authority, guidance, and wisdom are already here; they are available to us if we can just tune in to them. The only question then is, What is the best way to tap into this counsel? The mystics have been telling us for centuries, of course, that the best way to tap into God is through the silence of meditation. By placing your attention on God, and making your intention to follow the plan of God, everything you need will be added to you. That's what Jesus meant when he said, "Seek first the kingdom of God and His righteousness, and all these things shall be yours as well" (Matt. 6:33). Seek first God's counsel, God's wisdom, God's guidance, and everything else you need will be added.

Years ago, I thought I understood that passage, but I had it all wrong. Seeking the kingdom was usually said to mean joining the right church. If you sought first the kingdom of God by way of this church's teaching, then everything else you needed to live life would be found there. That is only half true. What you need is already present, but you have to do the work to tap into it. You have to have enough trust in yourself to believe that when these thoughts come to you, you will act on them. As foolish as this intuitive awareness may seem to the world, when you act on it everything falls into place.

"Your will is throughout the earth even as it is throughout the universe." I prefer to say "throughout the universe" rather than "in heaven" because of our association of heaven as a place where God dwells with the angels. That's not what heaven means. It means the universe, the stars, the planets. What keeps all those heavenly bodies from smashing into each other if not the will of God?

And so, what is the will of the Daddy? Is it complex or hard to discern? Is it to bring suffering to humanity to help us grow spiritually? In the Gospel of Luke, Jesus announces his agenda when he reads in the synagogue from the Book of Isaiah (61:1–2): "The Spirit of the Lord God is upon me, for He has anointed me to bring the good news to the afflicted. He has sent me to proclaim liberty to captives, sight to the blind, to let the oppressed go free, to proclaim a year of favor from the Lord." Then Jesus hands the scroll back to the attendant and says, "Today this scripture has been fulfilled in your hearing" (Luke 4:18–21). He is clearly stating his agenda, yet he makes no mention of suffering. Instead he talks of the "year of favor," the jubilee year when religious Jews were expected to forgive all debts owed to them. Does this sound like the message of a punishing Father who wants His children to learn by suffering?

The eighth chapter of the Gospel of Matthew begins with an account of Jesus being approached by a leper who says, "Lord, if you want to, you can make me clean." And Jesus says, "I want to; be clean." This is another clear expression of the will of God. Jesus doesn't have to think about whether to heal or not. He can know the very thoughts of God and act on them instantaneously. Once again, there is no sense that the leper should continue to suffer.

"You give us this day our daily bread." Our daily bread means everything we need in the form of what "prosperity" signifies. To prosper means to flourish in all areas of our lives, and to flourish abundantly. The will of God is for us to flourish abundantly in our financial situation, our career, our relationships, our social life. God wants us to enjoy and celebrate life.

Jesus taught that the kingdom of God is within, meaning that you don't need to go to priests and scribes for counsel and advice. So the next time you have a question about life, spend a few moments in silence and deposit that question as a seed in the fertile ground of the Holy Spirit, where all things are possible. We often believe that we can't accomplish something, and as a result we don't. We go only as far as our beliefs will allow us to go.

The Aramaic word Jesus used for bread, *lakhma,* includes all material things. Jesus is implying that we can bring things into reality by our intention and attention. That is the real meaning of faith or what Jesus referred to as "the single eye" (Matt. 6:22). When you focus with a single eye, you put your whole attention on something. Attention is the field of all possibilities and your intention is the seed you throw into that field and watch grow. The seed might be health, wealth, or good relationships, or it might be to pay your bills. But you must have an intention—the focus of your thought life and your spiritual life—and that intention to reap a bounty of good must be built on a foundation of truth. The truth is that God is for us, not against us, as it says in the Book of Jeremiah: "For I know the plans I have for you, says the Lord, plans for good and not for evil, to give you a future and a hope" (29:11).

One of the greatest truths uttered by any mystic was spoken by Jesus when he said to the people of his day (as well as to us in our day), "You are the salt of the earth," and likened them to "the light of the world" and "a city set on the hill" (Matt. 5:13–14). What he wanted the people to recognize was the exalted way God sees his children. When we get that truth into our being, our life is transformed and we move into an expanded consciousness, a Christ consciousness. And no religion has a monopoly on the Christ nature.

Not only does the Father give us every material need, but He also gives us the understanding to bring abundance into our own lives. Our Daddy, the great I AM, is the source of every good. The divine Presence may manifest as certain principles in the universe that have been here since the beginning of time. One of those eternal laws is simply stated as Give and you shall receive. Physicists might say, For every action there is an equal and opposite reaction; the ancient Hindus knew this as karma, or the law of cause and effect; in this century we say, Go with the flow. Simply put, if we want God to send us things, we can't hoard what we have. If your prayers are not working and you are struggling to make ends meet or to get where you want to go, I would seriously suggest that you look in your closets. If you have clothes in your closet that you haven't worn or even looked at for years, give them away, because you are blocking the flow. You have become a Dead Sea. If things flow into you but nothing flows out of you, you become stagnant. If you want the flow to continue coming in, you have to open up the dam. Everything is in flux, yet we try to stand still and fight the current. But if we have faith when we say to God, "You give us our daily needs," then we have no desire to hold on to everything because we know there's always more where that came from. Deepak Chopra tells the story of the time his former guru Maharishi Mahesh Yogi was discussing a new project with a group of his followers. It was a big project and one of the people in the room asked Maharishi where the money would come from to pay for the work. Without blinking, Maharishi answered, "From wherever it is at the moment."

We don't like to hear that we have to let go in order to receive. We would rather blame God and say that maybe God doesn't want to bless us. God always wants to bless. So it is up to us to put back into circulation what we have hoarded and what we continue to hoard. If for some reason I keep stuff that I'm not using, that literally says to the universe that I have a fearful spirit, a poverty mentality. I'm afraid I will never have enough, so the universe responds by saying, "Right, you will never have enough because that is your focus." Our thoughts of lacking enough are fears that set up a vibration that attracts to us the very thing we fear.

"You forgive us our offenses as we forgive our offenders." The Aramaic word *shbakn,* which we translate as "forgive," also means "to set free," "to release or untie." God frees us from our offenses to the same degree that we have freed our offenders—another configuration of the law of cause and effect. It means that if we want to be free, we no longer can be plugged into negative thoughts about a situation or person. If we release them, we in turn are empowered to start on a new path in life. What Jesus says here is that our forgiveness of others is the key that opens the floodgate of God's forgiveness. As *A Course in Miracles* and teachers like Caroline Myss have emphasized, we cannot progress without first forgiving not only those who have harmed us but also ourselves. In fact, God has already released us from the karmic effects of our wrongdoings, provided we have released others for their negative actions against us. Knowing this to be the truth, we are then able to allow that phrase to work directly on the negatively destructive emotion of the guilt we experience, whether real or imaginary. God does not want to judge us; he wants to forgive us and heal us.

"And you do not let us enter into the illusion of materialism, but you separate us from error." The phrase "Lead us not into temptation" always gave me fits. Even as a devout Catholic and a priest, I couldn't understand why we would have to beg God not to tempt us to do evil, as the language implies. What the original Aramaic actually means, however, is that God will never tempt anyone to put their focus entirely on the external. As good as all the wonderful things of the world may be, whether it's the food we eat or the clothes we wear, we cannot put our focus on that as our goal. We are reminded by Jesus that God does not tempt us to be "fooled" by matter, but separates us from the error of being material-minded instead of spirit-minded. Having fallen short of God's glory (being Spirit), we are often filled with resentment and bitterness. Emphasizing the words "you let us not enter into materialism" or "you keep us from the temptation of false appearances" heals and dissolves the bitterness that often accompanies the guilt we transfer to others as anger, and breaks the hold these negative past actions have continued to have on us on the level of our inner being.

The question of assigning the proper role to the material realm often confounds people, but it need not. Saint Paul never said, "Money is the root of all evil." He said, "The love of money is the root of all evil." The problem is not matter but putting all your focus on matter. We do the same thing with religion: we put our focus on rules even though Jesus kept putting his focus on spirit. Why not focus instead on what money is created from? Money is created out of the same substance from which we are all created: energy.

Jesus did not say, "Deliver us from evil" (or from "the evil one" as some translations have it). He said that the Father separates us from error, the error being the illusion of matter.

The Aramaic conclusion to the Lord's Prayer reads, "Because yours are the kingdom, the power, and the song throughout all ages, sealed in faith, trust, and truth." I take that to mean "You,

Daddy, make possible for me, your child, the abundant way of life because you've got it all. You have what it takes to provide for us and to this I say Amen." The Hebrew word *amen* comes from the Aramaic word *amena,* which means "faithful" or "truthful" or, more colloquially, "I back up this truth." The word was used in Jesus' day for making an oral agreement in lieu of a written contract. When Jesus said to his disciples, "Amen, Amen, I say unto you," he was saying, in effect, "Listen here, I'm going to tell you the truth, and I'll stand behind it." Think of that when you pray. At the end of your prayer, instead of just of tacking on the word "Amen," literally say, "Amen, God is faithful to this."

The Lord's Prayer teaches us that God is a good God who desires our abundance, peace, and prosperity. To this I can say Amen, meaning that God is faithful to that truth. God will always provide, and if for some reason the provision isn't there, then the problem is not on God's end. The problem is that we don't understand God as Jesus did. In saying Amen, we are acknowledging our responsibility in this faithful contract made between God and His children.

MEDITATION RITUAL ON THE LORD'S PRAYER

Especially for those of us who were raised as Christians, the Our Father has become a prayer that we rattle off almost like a mantra with no thought for what it is meant to convey. We have memorized the words but have long since lost any sense of their spiritual impact. An excellent way to say the Our Father after reading this chapter is to say it slowly, one phrase at a time, and meditate on each phrase and what it means. You could easily spend twenty minutes or more with the Lord's Prayer this way, saying it just a single time.

The following exercise and prayers can be used to prepare for your meditation on the Lord's Prayer, or in conclusion, or both.

Take three deep breaths as you begin to enter into the presence of God and become aware of His Holy Spirit, the Spirit that fills the whole universe and permeates every part of our being. As we open to that Spirit, we experience a rise in consciousness, an awareness of a deep sense of peace. Our God is not only with us but our God is in us and for us. And in that awareness a joy begins to well up as we experience not only the love of God but also the power of God. Experiencing that love is like being in a cooling mist that refreshes every part of our being and personality, our soul, spirit, and body. Now pray:

Lord, as we learn to pray as Jesus taught us, we begin to experience a supernatural energizing. We may not be able to understand it yet, but we do know that something new and refreshing is happening. Our relationship with you is becoming more intimate. There seems to be a freshness in the total environment in which we find ourselves, and because of it fear begins to diminish. As fear diminishes, so do the stresses that accompany it. Lord, we are open to your peace and your presence. We fully embrace your Spirit and we immerse ourselves into that Spirit as if we were immersing ourselves in water—sacred, supernatural water that refreshes and renews, heals and makes whole. And for this we thank you.

Lord, thank you for reshaping our lives and showing us through this prayer that our destiny is one of abundance. As we tune in to your voice, as we tune in to your will and your plan, our compass is reconnected and we stop going south when we should be going north. As we do so, Lord, we find the fulfillment we need without all the struggle that has caused us so much difficulty in the past. So be it. All is in harmony.

Father, you have opened up our consciousness to a more expansive awareness of your love, your presence, your whole being. You have helped us develop true communion and connection with you, so that in times of fear we begin to understand the needlessness of being in terror.

As we look to you, Lord God, in the manner in which Jesus taught us to look to you, we can see that you are all-powerful, all-knowing, everywhere present. Lord, you are almighty and you are all-loving and your desire is to consume us in the fires of your love. We have become aware that your advice, counsel, and wisdom are always available as we tune in. We tune in best to the prayer of silence we call meditation.

Your will is already present throughout the earth as it is throughout the universe, where absolute order reigns. Your will can be seen in the laws of the universe, the principles that guide every creative action with order and harmony. You give us everything we need to experience wholeness in our life. This is the bread you give us that as we gaze at nature, as we walk in the forest or near the water, or sit by a pond and give it our full attention, we begin to sense not only the beauty of that moment but also a powerful, all-consuming love emanating from that moment. We feel energized, never to be the same again.

Father, you forgive us all of our offenses; all we need to do is be aware of our willingness to forgive others the offenses they might have performed against us. Literally we put them in your light and release them with the awareness of Jesus' final prayer: Father, they did not know what they were doing. And because of this, Lord, such a clarity comes to our thinking and our awareness that we recognize that matter can no longer delude us. We cannot be tempted to put our whole focus, the single eye, upon only that which is matter, but rather we look down deep through that matter to experience your Spirit, the essence of our own being, for we truly are made in your image and we are Spirit.

And Father, to know that you do separate us and part us from all error helps us to realize that it is possible for us to trust you. You would not delude us. You are a Father who literally dances over his children who tune in to you, listen to you, love you, and are loved by you. Because of this, we are able to say that yours are the kingdom, the power, the song of praise of the universe from all ages throughout all ages, sealed with trust and in truth. To this, Lord, we say Amen.

HEALING SICKNESS AND SUFFERING

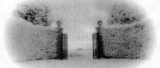

We have been taught that it is "the will of God" for us to suffer! . . .
We may believe that God wants us to be sick so that He may teach us
compassion and empathy. But this is not God's way of teaching us
compassion and empathy. . . . We bring misfortune upon our own
heads without the help of God. Hopefully, though, when our suffering
hurts badly enough, we will wake up to the error of our ways, and
change the causes which brought on our troubles.

◆

RoCCO A. ERRICO, *THE ANCIENT ARAMAIC PRAYER OF JESUS*

I will with God that none of His Sons should suffer.
◆
A COURSE IN MIRACLES, TEXT (6.I.11.7)

Prayer and healing are connected in some obvious ways. We pray for healing, and prayer in and of itself can be a form of healing. But is there some other way in which they are interconnected at their very core? To answer that question, we may first have to examine some of the prevailing misconceptions about sickness, suffering, and the nature of healing.

Christianity, especially Catholic Christianity as taught today, implies that sickness and suffering make us better, as if they were natural components of the process of developing compassion. I'm not so sure about that. Suffering may help you know what it is to feel helpless and alone, but I do not believe that sickness is in any way a prerequisite for compassion or spiritual growth. Teresa of Ávila and Hildegard of Bingen both suffered illnesses early in their lives, but later healed themselves. Hildegard lived into her eighties, which in the thirteenth century was no mean feat. Her relative healthiness certainly did not impinge on her holiness.

Just as I don't believe that sickness is necessarily a sign of developing compassion, neither do I think it is a sign of bad karma. We do not get sick because of some evil we did in a previous lifetime, or because of an insufficiently positive mind-set in this lifetime. This amounts to what Joan Borysenko rightly calls "karmic fundamentalism." Borysenko, a biologist and psychologist who believes that we have the power to heal ourselves, points out that a complex of causes may contribute to illnesses like cancer and heart disease, of which our own tendency to be negative or to suppress our most heartfelt desires may amount to only a small portion. Our mind-set and the emotional residue of bad choices and disappointments earlier in life are only part of a mixture of elements, each of which plays some role. We also have to take into account,

Borysenko adds, our genetic predisposition, our environment, what we eat, and how we take care of ourselves. Walking around with a head full of negative, depressing thoughts and eating a lot of junk food may indeed make it difficult to maintain a state of glowing health, yet we probably all know of at least one certified curmudgeon who eats burgers and fries with abandon, drinks and smokes like a sailor, and has still managed to remain strong and healthy—depressingly so—beyond the age of eighty.

Trying to generalize about the cause of illness can be an exercise in foolishness in any event. Some very saintly men and women, for instance, suffered greatly in their lives. Three of the holiest men in India—Sri Ramakrishna, Ramana Maharshi, and Jiddu Krishnamurti—all died rather painful deaths from various forms of cancer. Yet we can look at other saintly figures and find no illness at all. Paramahansa Yogananda died in 1952 after concluding a speech at a banquet for the Indian ambassador, and according to the mortuary director of Forest Lawn, his body showed no sign of decay during the twenty days his casket remained open. The Buddha, as far as we know, was never sick a day in his life, except when he almost starved himself to death by fasting in his youth. Jesus died a very painful death, but there is no record in the Gospels of his ever having been sick. Bernie Siegel said years ago that if a thousand people are suffering with the same disease and one is cured, we ought to forget for the moment the nine hundred and ninety-nine who either have died or are still sick and find out why the one got well.

Some of the great Christian healers of the twentieth century present equally paradoxical histories. With all of the power of God moving through her to heal others, Kathryn Kuhlman died of an enlarged heart from which she had suffered for the last few years of her life. Nor was she always a great exemplar of psychological health; her biographer Jamie Buckingham in *Daughter of Destiny* acknowledges that Kuhlman was probably the most insecure healer who ever graced the earth. Aimee Semple McPherson was one of the most powerful healers of this century, yet her arthritis was so bad that when she would kneel down to lay hands on people, everybody could hear her joints cracking. She ultimately died of an accidental overdose of painkillers at the age of fifty-four.

The healer Agnes Sanford, whom I knew personally, did not die of any illness. She said good-bye to her secretary, walked upstairs, sat down in a chair, and quietly went. Smith Wigglesworth, an English evangelist and healer who developed an international ministry in the 1920s and '30s, was a physically imposing man who worked as a plumber until his healing ministry took off. He refused to have medication or surgery, even when a case of appendicitis almost killed him early in his career. At the age of seventy, he suffered a continuing ordeal with kidney stones that lasted six years, but was never sick again until he died in 1947 at the age of eighty-seven.

To me, the only lesson to be gleaned from studying the lives of healers and holy people is that there is absolutely no correlation between holiness and sickness. I can find no reason to believe that we are not entitled to health and happiness as part of our spiritual life. When the concept that we create our own reality first began to appear some years ago, it was liberating, because it held out the possibility that we no longer had to view ourselves as the helpless victims of circumstance or of forces completely beyond our control. Now, however, it has become a kind of spiritual cliché that is accepted unthinkingly and applied in ways that are not helpful. If we create our own reality, this belief goes, then we are somehow responsible for all the bad things that happen to us. That can very easily be turned into a judgment against us whenever we become ill or suffer some misfortune. In an account of a sexual assault that appeared in *The New York Times* a few years ago, the assailant reportedly told the woman, as he was dragging her into the bushes of a park in Upper Manhattan, that she should examine her life to determine what she had done to deserve what was now happening to her. That's an extreme example of how the concept of creating one's own reality can be turned against us, but to my mind it is a direct outgrowth of the belief.

In one way, of course, we do create our own reality. If we see our reality connected with the Reality of God, and we see the love and mercy and presence of God as who we are, then we may more readily create a divine reality within ourselves. If we surround ourselves with prayer and meditation and images of the Divine, we are probably more likely to maintain an awareness of the Divine than if we immerse ourselves in violent fantasies. Do not be misled by misguided people who try to tell you that you are sick because you have the wrong mind-set, that you have created your own disease because you have done things that made you unhappy earlier in life, or because you did something regrettable in a past life. To begin with, the idea that we create our own reality comes from a misunderstanding of what reality is. Reality is the spiritual dimension. Reality is what Saint Paul means when he refers to being transformed by the renewal of our thinking. Most people nowadays take that to mean "positive thinking," but Paul meant it as transformation or metamorphosis, the caterpillar becoming the butterfly. No amount of positive thinking in the world can bring about that kind of transformation.

The Buddhist and Hindu understanding of reincarnation and karma are much more complex than most people care to discover. In the Buddhist conception, for instance, we don't reincarnate as some kind of permanent soul with a whole laundry list of good and bad deeds to account for. We merely carry with us certain tendencies, which both Hindus and Buddhists refer to as *samskaras* (a Sanskrit word that means "impressions" or "consequences"). In the broadest sense, the quality of these tendencies then conditions the new consciousness that arises through them and that brings about the existence of a new person in the process of rebirth. That's a far cry from saying that the pancreatic cancer with which you've just been diagnosed is the result of having been a member of the Gestapo in your last life! Such statements seek to imbue us with guilt that is not only unnecessary but powerfully counterproductive. We need to question such popular assumptions every bit as much as we question the dogmas of organized religion, whether Christianity, Islam, or Buddhism.

Everyone will suffer in some way or another. The Tibetan Buddhist teacher Sogyal Rinpoche likes to say that it's a mistake to look at others and assume that they have it easier than you do. There is poor people's suffering, he says, and rich people's suffering. Like sickness, suffering can be a sacred event. It can be used to repair the damage done on the spiritual level by negativity. But it is not the same as sickness. Christ and the Buddha both suffered in different ways. However, their suffering was not something negative. As I see it, the cross is a plus sign. From an energetic viewpoint, it is a magnifying glass in which all the scattered energies of the universe were brought to one point and intensified. Death on the cross was a sacred, loving act whose tremendous force is implied by all of the power that was released by Christ's death: the earthquake, the graves opening up, the Temple curtain being torn. Whether those events actually occurred as recorded in the Gospels is beside the point. They refer to the most powerful form of energy release that has ever been recorded. That is an indication of what God's love does.

I do not accept the theology that Jesus was sent here to die, because that makes God the Father look exceptionally cruel. I believe that Jesus' mission was to say that there is something beyond suffering and that the spirit does not die. Jesus' mission was the healing of fear. Saint Paul says that the last enemy to be conquered is death, because that is our greatest fear. All fear is essentially fear of separation, and in our minds, death is the ultimate separation.

The English word "sacrifice" comes from the Latin words *sacrum* and *facere,* which mean literally "to make sacred." Padre Pio, who lived in the first half of this century, suffered greatly in his life. He received the stigmata—bodily wounds representative of Christ's passion, most often on the hands, feet, and side, where the body of Jesus was pierced. Although Pio bled from the wounds, he never showed the symptoms of blood loss, and he was blessed with mystical abilities including bilocation, the power to be physically present in two places at the same time. Like the Polish visionary Sister Faustina, he saw suffering as an opportunity to change the negative current in consciousness to a positive one. Catholics used to refer to this as "reparation," meaning the repair of damage done in the spiritual realm. The concept of living simultaneously in different realms is a difficult one for many people to understand, even though we do lip service to the ancient spiritual principle of "As above, so below." In the Lord's Prayer, we say "on earth, as it is in heaven." Saint Paul said we do not fight against flesh and blood, but against the principalities and powers, a reference to spiritual energies that are creating havoc in the universe (Eph. 6). Prayer and fasting, the purpose of which is to focus on God, are two ways to help repair the damage on that level. According to the spiritual law, as we repair damage on the spiritual level, the natural world begins to be repaired at the same time.

Now let's take this idea a step further. From the perspective of energy medicine, thoughts can be good or bad; they can create something positive or something negative. The random violence that appears to be plaguing our country today is produced in the atmosphere around us. When Cain killed Abel, the earth cried out against the spilling of blood. That isn't just poetic speech; that is reality. In old mythological talk, they referred to angels and devils fighting, which was a way of saying that spiritual energies were in conflict. The Greek word usually translated as "demon" is *daimones,* which means "spirit energies" and can refer to either positive or negative energies. I don't believe in the Devil or devils as entities from hell, but I do believe that there are spiritual energies that can confuse, debilitate, depress, and make us sick. If I'm weak in my thinking and I walk into a crowd of negative thinkers, I may come away as miserable as they are. But if I'm working on who I am in God's sight through prayer and meditation, I have the power to change the whole crowd. If I change the spiritual dimension, the natural dimension will fall in line. Jesus said that whenever two or more are gathered in his name—meaning with his understanding, his commitment to God—they have a great amount of power to change things swiftly. This calls to mind a verse from the Old Testament in which God says to Moses that if the people keep His commandments, "Five of you shall chase a hundred, and a hundred of you shall chase ten thousand" (Lev. 26:8). I wonder what would have happened by now if people in cloistered monasteries or convents around the globe hadn't been praying all these years. Not one political pundit on earth expected the Berlin Wall to come down, and neither did I. Yet I believe it came down because a spiritual power had been released.

Some point to the ethnic strife in the Balkans as a sign that the world's consciousness has not changed, but I see it as a different kind of energy at work, and that is the negative energy generated by the failure to forgive. In the New Testament, Jesus says, "You will hear of wars and rumors of wars . . . and nation will rise against nation." But the Greek word translated as "nation" here is *ethnos,* which means "ethnic group." Medjugorje is right in the middle of Bosnia Herzegovina yet it has been spared all the bloodshed that swirled around it, perhaps because the people prayed. Even in an area where the mass consciousness is negative, what happens to others does not necessarily have to happen to you. Psalm 91 says,

A thousand may fall at your side,
ten thousand at your right hand;
but it will not come near you. . . .
Because you have made the Lord your refuge,
the Most High your habitation,
no evil shall befall you.

People often raise the question of why one person is healed and not another, which is also the subject of a book by Caroline Myss and Norman Shealy called *The Creation of Health*. Myss and Shealy posed some fascinating answers to this question, but at the end of the day I come away feeling much the way I do about why people get sick in the first place: It simply isn't always possible to ascribe the result to a single reason. I can't explain why healing occurs to one person in the pew and not to the one sitting next to her. I just know that it does happen. The healer Kathryn Kuhlman went to her grave saying, in effect, "I don't know why this works, other than to say that God is merciful."

I do happen to agree with one of the reasons Myss has posited: on a deeper level, some people don't *want* to be healed. They may be getting more attention from their spouse or friends than they ever got before, and they may not be ready to give that up even if the final payoff is death. When I was first doing my healing services at the church, members of my staff used to question me afterward, asking, "Why do you touch some, but you walk right by others?" I know when I stand in front of some people that they don't want to be healed. If I said to their faces that they didn't want to be healed, they would insist that I was wrong, but I just know this. I have also seen cases in which the person who is healed possesses none of the characteristics that many fundamentalists insist are prerequisites to healing. I have seen people restored, made whole, and cured instantly who did not seem to have great faith, and who did not appear to change their life to one of moral perfection. To paraphrase one of Kathryn Kuhlman's favorite statements, "Every time I get my theology straight, the Holy Spirit comes along and messes it up."

Believers and nonbelievers like to engage in endless debates on the subject of plane crashes or other calamities in which some people survive. The believers say that God was merciful in sparing the lives of the survivors. The nonbelievers say that's nonsense because if God is merciful, why did He let the rest of the passengers die? I prefer to phrase the issue in terms of the people who didn't get on the flight in the first place. They sometimes say, "At the last minute I had a feeling not to get on." In that sense, God is always extending His mercy and His wisdom, but only the person who is receptive and is not afraid to take the risk of looking and feeling stupid can avail himself of that mercy and wisdom. I was in Malibu just after one of those horrible fires in which every home in a certain section of the area was destroyed except one. The roof of this home wasn't even singed, but the people inside were very matter-of-fact about it. When a television reporter asked them what they had been doing during the fire, they said, "Praying." Everything around them was burned to the ground. Maybe other people were praying and their houses burned, but there it is.

How do you explain the priests in Hiroshima whose church was at ground zero when the atomic bomb was dropped? The church was demolished, but the rectory was spared and none of the priests suffered from radiation sickness. That is historical fact. Pious Catholics might say that they were saved because they were praying the rosary. Does that mean they wouldn't have been saved if they had been reciting the Psalms, or the Quran, or the Lotus Sutra? I don't know how to explain these things.

Events like the ones I've mentioned here—we could easily compile hundreds more—make God look capricious, but there is nothing capricious about the way things happen. I believe that much of the reason one person is healed and not another has to do with receptivity and faith on the part of each individual.

It should not surprise us that these are the same principles necessary for successful prayer. Receptivity and surrender go hand in hand, and that is where the irony, along with some of our difficulty in understanding this issue, may lie. Surrendering—being receptive—to God's will may at times mean that we do not immediately get well. This flies in the face of our rather simplistic notions of what constitutes health and sickness, and what suffering and healing mean. Agnes Sanford expressed the complexity of this question rather eloquently in her autobiography, *Sealed Orders*. "I learned to pray for my real desire," she wrote,

> to fix my attention on the wholeness that I wanted for myself or for someone else, and not to refuse any temporary symptoms that God through nature might use in order to bring about that wholeness. I learned to say, "This pain (or that discomfort) is just God's power working in me toward health and life, and as soon as it has accomplished what the body is trying to do, it will go away." I learned also to pass on this attitude toward pain or discomfort to other people for whom I prayed. If someone would call me up and say, "Since you prayed for my knee it hurts more than ever! It's terrible!" I would reply, "Don't lose your nerve. This pain is only the body calling together all its energies in order to heal. Bless it and give thanks for it, and it will pass." And so it would.

There have been times in my own life when I asked for illness or suffering to be taken away, and it did not disappear. What was I to make of that? My conclusion, which I realize may not satisfy everyone, is that perhaps the pain was a call for me to immerse myself more fully in the illness or suffering to understand what needed to be healed on a deeper level—on the level of soul or spirit. To do that can require a supreme act of surrender, of remaining receptive to God's thoughts and will for us in the most exacting of circumstances. We all tend to run from pain without asking why the pain is speaking to us in the first place. The most obvious example may be the business executive who is under too much pressure and develops ulcers. He wants surgery or medication to relieve the ulcers because he doesn't want to have to reexamine the high-pressure, fast-track style of life he has embraced. The modern spiritual healer Elizabeth K. Stratton addresses precisely this point in her book *Touching Spirit:*

> When someone comes to see me about a physical illness, my goal is to see their soul and the way it is trying to speak through their body. Illness breaks down the hold of the ego and allows the soul to shine through. This experience is not always pleasant and is often frightening to us. We don't like being out of control. Most of us reach for the remedy that will put us back in control as quickly as possible: pain medication, antidepressants, antibiotics, cold remedies, surgery. . . . The trouble with this approach is that in putting our ego back in control, we are ignoring what our soul is trying to tell us. Then the soul has to find another way to get us to pay attention. Each time it tries and fails, it becomes more insistent, more forceful. Maybe another illness is created, or an accident takes place, or nightmares occur. The cycle starts all over again, until we can break it by paying attention to the soul.

Stratton later quotes the words of Jesus from the Gnostic Gospel of Thomas: "If you bring forth what is within you, what you bring forth will save you. If you do not bring forth what is within you, what you do not bring forth will destroy you." She goes on to say,

Illness is the soul's message to our conscious ego self that there is something more, something meaningful to be explored down in the center of the suffering. There is a pearl of wisdom, a nugget of gold to be found among the dross, the base metal, the *prima materia* of the body. Like in statues of Kali, there is a small golden goddess of spiritual rebirth in the belly of suffering. This is the alchemical process of healing, as if base metal were being turned to gold. This is the resurrection process that we are all engaged in. Instead of rising above our pain, we need to dive down into the center of it, distill out the true meaning it has for our life, and allow this meaning to heal us.

And so the notion that sickness or disease is the result of a negative mind-set or a kind of punishment for having lived inappropriately is wrong primarily because it puts the emphasis in the wrong place. Illness can be seen not as a judgment on us but as a challenge or a call to examine our lives, reevaluate what we are doing, and possibly change direction. On the most practical level, an illness can lead us to change our diet, reduce the level of stress in our life, or find work that is more congruent with who we are. But to hear that call and respond appropriately, we need to remain as receptive to the thoughts of God as we do in authentic prayer.

Remaining receptive to the message of suffering—whether it manifests as a physical malady or some form of psychological torment or confusion—is often the last thing we want to do. I had gotten to the point in my healing ministry where, despite the great success I was having, I had begun to see people as merely objects to be healed. I didn't have time to see them as individuals. There followed a period of struggle during which I began to doubt my own ability and worthiness; at the same time, I began to get sick. Yet my ministry was providing me with both a sense of great personal accomplishment and the financial wherewithal to become independent of the church. Abandoning it was not an idea that I would welcome gratefully, or even entertain, for that matter.

The year was 1990 and I had just finished a healing service at the Anaheim Convention Center. I may have looked to the rest of the world like a highly successful healer, but I could already sense my own energy dropping and I was beginning to feel depleted and uninspired. The previous year I had become so exhausted by people literally attacking me at healing services that I had to request the conference coordinator to supply guards to take me to the podium. If that sounds like the action of a cult leader, at times it felt that way to me, too. On one level, all the commotion was exciting. That night in Anaheim, the police had to turn away three thousand people, and during the service the stage was littered with twenty wheelchairs left there by people who were healed. It was an exciting time—and yet I felt as if I wasn't there.

My associate Paul Funfsinn was standing near the platform, because he always stays very close to me in case I need something. I turned to him and said very deliberately, "Look around. This is over."

"What do you mean?" he said.

"I can't do this anymore," I said.

The conference coordinator had already said he wanted to sign me up for next year. I looked at him and repeated what I'd just said to Paul: "I can't do this anymore." I knew in my heart something wasn't right, although I didn't know what it was. Now I see that I had become object-oriented. I seemed to have lost my personal life.

The next couple of years were filled with bouts of self-doubt and mental anguish. After two or three years of suffering and sickness, I came to the realization that I was pretty much like all those people I had been helping to heal. I certainly knew I wasn't healing them, that I was just a channel for God's healing work. But even when you know that in your bones, it can still be difficult not to feel a little self-important, or at least to feel that those people are not so important. Eventually I was led to work with people who wanted to come to my house, and I've since learned how to handle private sessions or talking with people for spiritual consultation over the phone. I have been far happier working in this way and conducting healing workshops for a few hundred rather than services for thousands.

I wasn't especially eager to hear God's message in all this, and you could probably say that I was dragged kicking and screaming into my own liberation. But by listening to that inner voice in the worst of times, I feel that I've been able to make it through to the best of times. All God asks of me is that I remember that I'm an expression of God. If I can keep solidly in my head the understanding that He is appearing through me, then I can do what I am supposed to do in bringing God to the wounded. Since God is the One who cures, I don't take credit for the healings and I don't shoulder any blame for those who don't heal.

Whatever the reason for their not being healed, I know that it is finally between them and God.

Despite all these apparent incongruities, I still firmly believe that we are not supposed to be sick. I don't know yet why we get sick. I get sick myself, but I'm not the model, and when I do get sick that's not part of the perfect will and plan. I believe as Kathryn Kuhlman did that even if I don't get well, I must go to my grave believing that for me to be well is the perfect will. Gandhi said, "If I arrive at a point where I can no longer bring that presence of God to cure me, then write on my tombstone, 'Hypocrite.'" Like Gandhi, I believe there has to come a point in my life when sickness no longer exists for me.

I also believe that cellular memories that go all the way back to the time when we were just a light with God are trying desperately to come forth. But our belief system can stop them. If Jesus said that nothing is impossible, did he really mean that? Was he kidding people? I have to believe that those statements represent the essence of the spiritual energy that emanated from the Master. Our job—perhaps our only job—is to remain open and receptive to the message even when we least feel like it.

PRAYER READING FOR HEALING

For this prayer exercise, imagine that what you are reading is the voice of Jesus speaking to you in intimacy and in utter loving-kindness. Or you may want to imagine another image that gives you comfort, such as Mother Mary, Kuan Yin, Tara, Saint Francis of Assisi, the Buddha, or a loved one who has passed on. You may record the prayer on an audiotape (altering the wording in a few places if you have chosen another sacred figure) to play at various times throughout the day, including just before sleep. You may also wish to play some appropriate music in the background. I recommend the *Chant* and *Ave Maria* by the Benedictine monks of Santo Domingo de Silos; the Pachelbel Canon; or *Om Namaha Shivaya* by Robert Gass and On Wings of Song; but feel free to pick music of your own. Some nights when I meditate or pray, I just throw on one of my favorite CDs by Kenny G., either *Breathless* or *The Moment.*

> *"Behold I stand at the door and knock."*
> REVELATIONS 3:20

"It is true. I stand at the door of your heart, day and night. Even when you are not listening, even when you doubt it could be Me, I am there. I await even the smallest sign of your response, even the least whispered invitation that will allow Me to enter. And I want you to know that whenever you invite Me, I do come— always without fail, with infinite power and love, bringing the many gifts of My Spirit. I come with My mercy, with My desire to forgive and heal you, and with a love for you beyond your comprehension.

"I come longing to console you and give you strength, to lift you up and bind all your wounds. I bring you My light. I come with My power, with My grace, to touch your heart and transform your life. My peace I give to still your soul.

"I know you through and through. I have followed you through the years, and I have always loved you—even in your wanderings. I know every one of your problems. I know your needs and your worries. And yes, I know all of your mistakes.

"But I tell you again that I love you, and I have shed My blood to win you back. If you only ask Me with faith, My grace will touch all that needs changing in your life; I will give you the strength to free yourself from error and all its destructive power."

Now see Jesus or the figure you have chosen reaching out to you. Accept his love as he continues to speak to you:

"I know what is in your heart. I know your loneliness and all your hurts—the rejections, the judgments, the humiliations. I carried it all for you so you might share My strength and victory. I know especially your need for love, how you are thirsting to be loved and cherished.

"But how often have you thirsted in vain by seeking that love selfishly, striving to fill the emptiness inside you with passing pleasures. Do you thirst for love? Come to Me all you who thirst. I will satisfy you and fill you.

"*I thirst for you.* I thirst to love you and to be loved by you. Come to Me, and I will fill your heart and heal your wounds. I will make you a new creation, and give you peace, even in your trials.

"*I thirst for you.* You must never doubt My mercy, My desire to forgive, My longing to bless you and live My life in you. *I thirst for you.* Thirst for Me. Give Me your life—and I will prove to you how important you are to My Heart.

"Trust in Me. Ask Me every day to enter and take charge of your life, and I will. I promise you before My Father in heaven that I will work miracles in your life. Why would I do this? Because *I thirst for you.* All I ask of you is that you entrust yourself to Me completely. I will do all the rest.

"All that you have sought outside of Me has only left you more empty, so do not cling to the things of this life. There is nothing I cannot forgive and heal, so come now, and unburden your soul.

"There is one thing I want you to remember always, one thing that will never change: *I thirst for you*, just as you are. It is your belief in My love that will change you.

"Look at the cross, look at My heart that was pierced for you. Have you not understood My cross? Then listen again to the words I spoke there, for they tell you clearly why I endured all this for you: '*I thirst . . .*' (John 19:28).

"Yes, I thirst for you. You have tried many other things in your search for happiness: why not try opening your heart to Me, right now, more than you ever have before.

"Come to Me with your misery, with your troubles and needs, and with all your longing to be loved. I stand at the door of your heart and knock. . . . Open to Me, for *I thirst for you.*"

Let us now, with humble hearts, go to Jesus and receive His Divine mercy.

Take three deep breaths, be quiet for a few moments, and then express your gratitude to God for His healing, loving mercy in any way that is comfortable for you. Sense yourself clothed fully in light, allowing that light to touch the areas of your life or body needing renewed health. Then slowly open your eyes.

THE FIVE STAGES OF HEALING TOWARD WHOLENESS

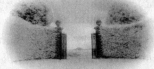

*The healing power of God moves through the spiritual body of man
into his physical body, and this understanding helped tremendously
in my prayer for healing, either for myself or others.*

◆

AGNES SANFORD, *SEALED ORDERS*

*It was evident in all miracles performed by Lahiri Mahasaya that
he never allowed the ego-principle to consider itself a causative force.
By the perfection of his surrender to the Prime Healing Power,
the master enabled It to flow freely through him.*

◆

PARAMAHANSA YOGANANDA, *AUTOBIOGRAPHY OF A YOGI*

In the time of Jesus, the Jews believed that under the proper circumstances the pool at Bethesda possessed healing powers. "At certain seasons," according to the Gospel of John, an angel of the Lord would roil the waters, and the first one into the pool after this event would be healed of all infirmities. Invalids, including the blind and the lame, gathered around the pool waiting for the waters to ripple. When Jesus visited the pool at Bethesda, an invalid of thirty-eight years was lying nearby waiting for the angel to trouble the waters (John 5). Approaching the unfortunate man, Jesus asked him, "Do you want to be made whole?"

This question suggests more than a simple healing of the part of his body that was diseased; it suggests an integration of all elements of his being. But the invalid responded with an excuse, while pointing a finger of blame toward the others gathered near the pool. "Sir, I have no man to put me into the pool when the water is troubled," he said, "and while I am going, another steps down before me."

Ignoring the sick man's negative attitude, Jesus said in an authoritative voice, "Get up. Pick up your mat and go home." Instantly the man was cured! What happened?

I believe that this scenario is presented as a message to the healer more than to those needing to be healed. Jesus did not scold the man to "have faith" as so many well-intentioned evangelists and faith healers of the TV variety so often do. (On some occasions, Jesus did rather forcibly question his disciples' faith, but they had been with him so long that he held them to a higher standard.) Knowing his connection with God and aware of the essence of his nature as light-energy, Jesus simply spoke from that place of authority within himself the words that set the invalid free of his paralysis.

From that place of authority rooted in unconditional love within, which Jesus always called "the kingdom," energy radiated like a spiritual laser beam and disintegrated the darkness that had paralyzed the man. This "invalidation," although evident in his body, had most likely first occurred in the man's spiritual or psychical being or both. Today we are increasingly aware of the interconnections among the spirit, mind, and body and the need to work toward integrating and harmonizing these three elements.

The story of the pool at Bethesda, however, implies that another force is at work in the healing process: Spirit energy. One of the most unfortunate developments in both the medical and religious establishments over the preceding centuries has been the dissection of the human being into three parts—body, mind, and spirit—each of which was assigned to the specialists trained to deal with only that part under their control. The body was shipped off to the medical doctor, the psyche (Greek for "soul," originally the vital principle, later simply the mind) was treated by a psychiatrist or psychotherapist, and the spirit by the clergyman. Sadly, each of these healers was on some level at odds with the others' approach to healing, having been taught that theirs was the one true path. As Dr. Larry Dossey has written, for example, medical doctors have generally been loath to invoke the spiritual in their healing practice, and have resisted the notion that prayer heals. All too often, religious teachers have ignored or played down the psychological implications of their teachings. And, at least until the recent resurgence of Jungian psychology, the therapeutic world has traditionally looked askance at anything spiritual.

Having practiced spiritual healing for over twenty-five years, I am convinced that the energy of God flowing to the human spirit is filtered through one's thoughts and beliefs and only then affects the physical body. Yet the full result of this energy may not be experienced in the body for some time. Because of this, the sick person needs the help of a spiritual healer along with other forms of medical treatment to increase the energy flow through his or her system. I would liken this effect to jump-starting a car. When the battery in a car does not have enough juice to start the engine, we call for someone to bring their jumper cables and hook up the dead battery to the battery of a car that has much more juice in it. Spiritual healers, as well as all healers who stay tuned in to the Source of this juice, have the necessary energy to jump-start another person. The way the spiritual healer stays in tune is through the act of prayer. This explains why so many people who attempt self-healing have a difficult time experiencing wellness. They need another individual who has more energy and knows how to release and project that energy to others.

There comes a time in all of our lives when we must ask ourselves, as Jesus asked the man at the pool of Bethesda, "Do I want to be whole?" If the answer is yes, the energy of God in the form of guidance and wisdom will flow in our direction. The most potent way I have found to experience this energy flow is through the practice of meditation as a connection with the light-energy of God. The energy that goes out during prayer is one that the human mind cannot comprehend but the human body can feel. We may also experience it on the soul level in the form of peace of mind. For this reason alone, prayer is spiritual therapy. It can produce an energy that aids the diagnosis of an illness through clairvoyance and clairaudience; can help cure the illness through the release of spiritual energy; and can relieve the pain of illness and preserve health.

If, as I have indicated, we often do not have enough spiritual energy to heal ourselves, and if, as has been my own personal experience, even healers sometimes have to turn to other spiritual heal-ers to be regenerated, what is the point of praying for healing at all? Isn't it an exercise in futility, and wouldn't our time be better spent simply seeking out a spiritual healer to pray for us? Not at all. Let's return for a moment to my metaphor of healing as jump-starting a car with a weak battery. We all know that it's possible for a battery to become so depleted of power that it cannot even be jump-started by a fully charged battery. In that instance, the dead battery doesn't respond at all and has to be replaced at much greater cost to the car's owner. At the very least, authentic prayer keeps your energy level alive and opens the channels for you to receive healing, whether it comes directly from God or through the intervention of a healer. Prayer prevents your internal levels from falling so low that reviving them becomes costly and arduous.

On another level, prayer experienced as loving communion with God brings an awareness that God is for us, not against us. Through prayer, we can come to know that events that seem to be tragic are not a judgment from God but have occurred for specific reasons. This in itself is uplifting and can facilitate and speed the healing process. When these apparently tragic or devastating events do happen, moreover, we can follow a process of healing toward wholeness that has been described and documented by mystics and students of mysticism such as Padre Pio and Evelyn Underhill. Drawing on their wisdom as verified by my own experience, I con-ceive of the healing process in five stages, each of which releases its own unique energy.

The first stage can be called the *awakening*. In this stage we allow ourselves the luxury of discovering the elegant spirit that resides in us all. The awakening stage can be particularly difficult for those whose self-worth has been devastated over the years. For these people to see themselves as "wondrously made" can be an impossible dream. Most of us have been taught to know ourselves as a physical body that is having a spiritual experience. In this stage, we come to grips with the truth that the human being is a spiritual entity temporarily having a physical experience. The awakening stage of the healing process begins when we decide that life has to consist of much more than we are currently experiencing. Both joy and pain are present in the awakening stage as they are throughout our whole life.

The next stage can be termed the *purification*. During this stage we remove from our life everything that we feel separates us from God. Energized by the new sense of power revealed in the first stage, we take responsibility for the change or transformation we desire in our lives. Prayer takes top priority in our attempt to do God's will in everything. One of the classic purifying events I experienced in my life occurred when I was still a parish priest and happened to be involved in an auto accident on a Los Angeles freeway. I was riding in my brand-new Ford Crown Victoria when I noticed that the traffic in front of me had come to a complete stop. As the person driving my car brought us to a safe stop, I watched in mounting horror while an 18-wheel tractor-trailer three lanes to our right attempted to stop, jackknifed, and began careening across all three lanes. With the inevitability of a freight train, the truck hit my car broadside.

I was lucky to escape with my life. There was shattered glass all over me, in my clothing, even in my underwear. I was hospitalized with minor injuries, but despite my apparently miraculous escape, I was consumed with anger and bitterness over this event. I was angry at the drivers in front of me who had stopped, and at the driver of the truck for totaling my new car. Over the course of a month, however, I was able to begin to forgive them. It wasn't easy and required a purification of my attachment to anger, vengefulness, and self-righteousness. And because I didn't fully learn the lesson of forgiveness at that time, I had to learn further lessons during the ensuing years.

Part of the process of healing toward wholeness requires the unplugging of one's thought-energy from past events and past hurts. This can be accomplished through the prayer of meditation whereby one places into the light of God the hurtful event along with people who are perceived as having caused one pain. Marianne Williamson, the popular interpreter of *A Course in Miracles,* has said that when she felt anger and resentment toward someone, she would constantly repeat to herself, "I forgive you (name), and I release you to the universe." After time, her angry, hurtful feelings would be dissolved and she could treat the person with equanimity. Christians may do much the same by envisioning the objects of their anger in the loving arms of Jesus, then releasing them to the light. Agnes Sanford called this "the healing of memories." The memories are retained but the sting that once accompanied them is dissolved. To confront these issues is a painful experience but the resulting freedom and joy are well worth the effort.

Following purification comes stage three, *illumination.* In the stage of illumination, we begin to perceive life through spiritual eyes and ears. On the practical level, we may describe this stage as an extended "Aha!" experience. Illumination in the form of revelation causes the illumined one to get a grasp on personal experience in a way that the logical mind has not been able to do. This can be highly energizing, for it brings with it feelings of hope and confidence and an awareness that there is more to life than what has been revealed by the five senses alone. Illumination is often accompanied by a sense of being connected with all of creation. This sense of connectedness is real and is not symbolic or fantasized. The illumination experience sheds light on the true nature of all life, which is energy. Our human nature as energy is not so much a fact we understand intellectually as one we experience. Once we know on an experiential level who and what we are, our being resonates to a higher vibration called love: love for God, for ourselves, for the land, for others. To injure or destroy another in any way then goes against our true nature, for to do so would cause injury to ourselves.

To deepen our awareness of our identity as a spiritual being, we proceed to the fourth stage of the healing process, called by many mystics *the dark night of the soul.* This stage has often been misunderstood by those who live only on the sense level and has occasionally been romanticized by those who have not actually experienced it. As described by John of the Cross and other mystics who have lived through it, the dark night is not merely a brief period of tortured soul-searching or despair that occurs sometime between the onset of the spiritual search and enlightenment. Someone for whom I was praying once said to me, "This has been the worst week of my life. I guess I'm in the dark night of the soul."

He thought the dark night was going to last only a week! Mine lasted nine and a half years. It is not a night but an epoch. But the beauty of it is that God strips away that which is *good.* The dark night, then, is not a time of complete despair but a period during which the individual is given the opportunity to make more rapid progress toward union with God. If, in the second stage, the individual purifies himself, then during the dark night of the soul God does the purifying. When God purifies, however, He is not removing from us anything that might be considered bad, evil, or sinful. God is actually purifying the good and better elements from our life so that we may experience the best, which is God Himself. God says, "I'm going to take away all this good stuff so you can have something *better.*" In my own case, I was enjoying a fairly secure life as a parish priest but I wasn't living up to my full potential as a spiritual teacher or being. I was being stymied by my bishop but I was fearful of risking change. God had to set me up in a sense by letting me experience being thwarted at what I wanted to do, which ultimately pushed me to go out on my own. I lost my security, but the end result is that I have been able to help thousands more people to heal, and in doing so to discover my real potential. In the process, I had the satisfaction of learning how to do a number of things that had previously been done for me. That was another example of God taking away something good in order to give me something better.

In his Letter to the Philippians, Saint Paul reminds the followers of Christ to focus the energies of their attention on that which is "excellent" (4:8). I interpret this to mean that we are called to fix our mind on the best gift offered us, which is God. By keeping our eyes on God as light-energy, the dark night is transformed into the brightness of day. (Eastern Orthodox mystics still refer to God as the "bright darkness.") At that point, the mystical union between the lover and the beloved takes place. All sense of insecurity and dependence on the ego begins to fade into nonexistence. We become one with the light, transfigured as Jesus was in the presence of his disciples on Mount Tabor, where his garment glowed with the radiance of sunlight. His inner being, his essence as light-energy, shone through his physical body and clothes, revealing for all time the experience of high-voltage vibration available to all God's children.

We all have inherent in us this potential to radiate divine energy, because we are "children of the light," children of the Spirit illuminated by a supernatural glow flowing from the fire of love itself, God. As we pass through the purification stage, we let go of all the unwanted things in our life, the things that we feel are keeping us from God. During the dark night of the soul, as God takes over the purification process, love and trust have an opportunity to grow and flourish as never before. As this occurs, we can more readily yield ourselves to God, knowing that He has our best interests at heart. In this act of surrender, God's Spirit takes over much more of our vessel, through which to function. When asked how he was able to bilocate, Padre Pio replied, "I don't know. I just told God that when He has need of me, to use me." That is genuine surrender.

In the act of being a yielded vessel, we open ourselves up to an unlimited energy. This indeed prepares us for entering the fifth stage of the healing process, called *mystical union*. In this stage, lover and beloved become one. On the spiritual level, God is the Lover who empowers His beloved with the ability to perform "miraculous" feats, an ability that springs from the unlimited love God has for all His creation. Through our openness to God and our willingness to be one with Him, we transcend our material body and live in the realm of spirit. This allows that energy of God's presence to manifest itself any way it chooses, knowing intuitively that it can reveal itself only as the energy of loving action.

Wholeness is achieved from the inside out, from the internal to the external level. In the five-stage process of healing toward wholeness, one concentrates on an internal transformation of consciousness that is able to affect the external realm. Anyone can receive a physical healing or cure and yet never experience the fullness of joy and inner peace that is available to all of us who give priority to the work of healing our psyche and spirit. Wholeness becomes a definite possibility, for with God and the energy of God's love, all things are possible.

Identifying the Stage of Your Healing Process

As you read through this chapter, you may have felt that you recognized one of the five stages in your own spiritual healing process. As I said in the Introduction, healing is a comprehensive practice that includes not only bodily ailments and diseases but also deep-seated psychological wounds and ongoing spiritual dilemmas. And so although the five stages I've outlined apply to a physical healing crisis, they can also be applied more generally to your overall spiritual development—your healing toward divine wholeness.

During your prayer and meditation time this week, remain open to God's voice in helping you discover what stage of the healing process you are in. You may actually find that more than one applies to you, and that is perfectly natural. Stages often overlap, and rarely is there a dramatic line of demarcation between one and the next. Simply try to get a feel for where you are, what you have accomplished spiritually in your life, and where you may be headed. But don't focus sharply on the future or begin to fear that you won't be able to deal with, say, the dark night of the soul. God provides the necessary strength and energy to take you through each stage of the journey as you need it, and projecting into the future can actually hold you back.

Keep in mind that every stage of healing toward wholeness has its own graces and difficulties, and accept where you are now as exactly the right and perfect place for you to be at this time. However, one element ties all five stages together, and that is a continuing growth in your love and compassion for others. The healing path of prayer, like any other authentic path, is ultimately based on love. As Jack Kornfield says in his book *A Path with Heart,* "All other spiritual teachings are in vain if we cannot love. Even the most exalted states and the most exceptional spiritual accomplishments are unimportant if we cannot be happy in the most basic and ordinary ways, if, with our hearts, we cannot touch one another and the life we have been given." You may find the following prayer helpful in opening your heart to allow love and mercy to flood in as you proceed on your journey.

Blessed Sister Faustina's Prayer of Mercy

Sister Faustina died in 1938 in a convent of the Congregation of Sisters of Our Lady of Mercy in Cracow, Poland. Born Helen Kowalska, she came from a poor farming family and had only three years of basic schooling. Seven years before her death, she experienced a vision of Jesus, clothed in a white garment, which she described in her diary:

> One hand was raised in blessing, the other was touching the garment at the breast. From the opening in the garment at the breast came forth two large rays, one red, and the other pale. In silence I gazed intently at the Lord; my soul was overwhelmed with fear, but also with great joy. After a while, Jesus said to me, "Paint an image according to the pattern you see, with the inscription: Jesus, I trust in You."

On another occasion, Jesus gave this explanation to Sister Faustina:

> The pale ray stands for the Water that makes souls righteous; the red ray stands for the Blood that is the life of souls. These two rays issued forth from the depths of my most tender mercy at that time when my agonizing heart was opened by a lance on the cross.

Before saying Sister's Faustina's prayer, you may say: "Lord, here I am. Use me in the manner you see fit that I may ever be what you have proposed for me to be—a light shining in the darkness to those who have lost hope from one cause or another."

SISTER FAUSTINA'S PRAYER

O Lord God, as many times as I breathe, as many times as my heart beats, as many times as my blood pulsates through my body, so many times do I want to glorify your mercy, your presence, your light. I want to be completely transformed into your light and mercy and to be your living reflection, your living energy, O Lord. May the greatest of all divine attributes, that of your unlimited mercy, pass through my heart and body to my neighbor.

Help me, O Lord, that my eyes may be merciful, so that I may never suspect or judge others by appearance.

Help me, O Lord, that my ears may be merciful, so that I may give heed to my neighbors' needs and not be indifferent to their pains and moaning.

Help me, O Lord, that my tongue may be merciful, so that I should never speak negatively of my neighbor but have a word of comfort and forgiveness for all.

Help me, O Lord, that my hands may be merciful and filled with good deeds, so that I may even take on the most toilsome task that belongs to others.

Help me, O Lord, that my feet may be merciful, so that I may hurry to assist my neighbor who is in need.

Help me, O Lord, that my heart may be merciful, so that I myself may feel the sufferings of my neighbor, thereby refusing my heart to no one, even those who will take advantage of my kindness.

O Lord God, let your light, let your mercy rest upon me. Amen.

CONGRUENCY IN PRAYER: LISTENING TO GOD AND FOLLOWING THROUGH

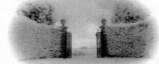

One of the greatest secrets that I have learned through the years is that when I have realized my own helplessness and have acknowledged it to Him, I have received some of the greatest manifestations of His power that I have ever experienced. You are nearest your possession of this imparted grace when you realize your own helplessness and your complete and entire dependence upon the Lord.

I am reminded of the young lady who, in describing faith, used this illustration. She said, "When I was learning to float on water, I realized I had to completely relax and without fear trust the water to hold me up—it worked. I floated—in the same way I faithed."

❖

KATHRYN KUHLMAN, *GOD CAN DO IT AGAIN*

There's an old story that you may have heard but that bears repeating, about a man stranded on the roof of his house during a raging flood. He prays to God to save him, and while he's praying he is approached by a series of rescue boats. As each boat comes near him, the man refuses to get in, proclaiming that God will save him. When he finally drowns and comes before the Lord, he asks why God did not answer his prayers and save him. "Who do you think," the Lord replies, "sent all those boats?"

The problem with our prayers sometimes is not just that we spend too much time asking God for favors, but that even when He responds we don't hear Him because we're expecting a different answer. Throughout this book I have tried to offer you a variety of ways to pray, but my gut feeling is that you can probably talk to God in just about any fashion as long as you maintain awareness. As you pray, remain alert to any response you may receive and be aware that the voice of God may come as a thought entering your head, a hunch, or an instinct. However the response comes, you need to consider it seriously and then act in congruency with it. What do I mean by that?

Living congruently with our prayer means that we cannot pray for something and act in a contrary way. As the Lord's Prayer makes explicit, if you pray for God to forgive you, you have to forgive the person you're holding a grudge against, too. And if you are going to pray for peace in the family, you need to know that God and the angels have a funny way of answering that kind of prayer. I imagine the dialogue going something like this:

"Oh, did you see Mabel pray for peace?"

"Yeah, she doesn't know the truth, does she?"

"No, she doesn't know that God is going to make *her* bring peace to the family."

You can't pray for peace in the family and expect God to let someone else bring it. If you pray for something, be aware that you probably will be the angel that delivers it in the physical realm. You must have congruency in what you think, in what you say, in what you feel in your heart, and in what you do. You have to follow your guidance, which may take the form of a sudden impulse to make a phone call or an urge to write a letter. When I started on this path, I had to take some big steps right at the beginning. One day I said to my bishop that I would like to feel more connected with the people. "I don't want to live in this rectory and have everything taken care of," I said bravely. "I'd like to get out, rent my own home, and take care of myself, because I can't really relate to people who say they don't have enough money to buy food for their children. I don't know what that feels like."

My desire to open my heart was innocent enough, but I wasn't at all prepared for the consequences. So I moved out and began to live on my own, which was fine at first. Then one day after praying, I decided to make breakfast. I went to the cupboard and was shocked to discover that hardly any food was left—a major crisis for me, since I love to eat. Then I went to the refrigerator and all I could find was something green that was growing in back. I was so used to being taken care of by the parish that I was a little like a teenager who moves out of his parents' house and doesn't realize he has to buy his own food and pay his own rent, and that it all requires money. I didn't know what else to do, so I immediately went to what I call my "prayer chair." That's the chair in the house where I go when I want to pray and I mean business. I sat down in that chair and I said, "Okay, God, look. I have done all this for you. Now the least you can do is supply me with the money to buy food."

I learned many years later that when you are talking with God or anyone else and you start to ask why, you don't want an answer. You want an argument. I was getting angry. "I need money to buy food," I said. "I don't know what I'm going to do. Please open up the door and give me guidance."

Stone silence. This went on for a while until finally a thought dropped into my head to go visit Sally, which was the last thing I wanted to do. Sally was the sad sack of the parish. I had been told that she got up in the morning, put on her bathrobe, and never took it off until evening. I could believe that because whenever I talked with her, all I heard was woe. "My life is so miserable," she would say. "I'm always sick. I can't breathe, and my heart is closing in."

It's tough to be a pastor sometimes because you are supposed to listen with a sympathetic ear. As much as you may be trying to do that, your feet want to get up and leave. So when this thought came into my mind, in my wisdom I replied, "No, I'm not going to visit Sally. I can't put up with that today. Lord, give me money to buy food."

Each time the thought returned to visit Sally, I rejected it. This went on for another half hour. Finally, because there was no other way, God dropped the next little seed of a thought into my head to go visit the local Lutheran pastor, who was a dear friend of mine and whose company I truly enjoyed.

Have you ever noticed that when God seems to say what is pleasing to you, you very quickly agree with Him? I got in my car, turned on the engine, and down the street I went. As it happens, Sally lived just a few blocks away from where I was living, on the way to the Lutheran church. When I got to her corner, the wheel seemed to turn in my hands and I found myself on her street and in her driveway, where I stopped. I thought, How can I be inconspicuous and back out of here? But at that moment, I saw the curtain being pulled back and there was Sally, looking out the window with a big smile on her face. I immediately thought, Now you've done it. She's seen me, and there's no escaping it.

When I went to the door, she greeted me all dressed up, with makeup on and a joyful look in her eye. She was excited about being alive, and for two hours I listened to her rattle on about all of the blessings that had come into her life the last few weeks. My God, I thought, this must be what conversion is all about. I didn't know which one of us had been converted, her or me, but I just listened and began to pick up some of her excitement. I felt so uplifted that I forgot why I had come out in the first place. As I got up to leave, Sally said, "Just a minute before you go. Come on in here, I've got something for you."

She led me into the kitchen. There on the table were several shopping bags, all filled with groceries. One big bag was packed with nothing but roasts and steaks. I couldn't believe my good fortune. I piled the bags into my car and went back home and unloaded everything, feeling very grateful. As I sat down to thank God, I heard a voice within me. I have never yet heard a voice "out there," and I would probably drop dead from fright if I did. But I do hear it internally, where it counts. The voice asked me, "Now, what's the lesson you've learned?"

God had never talked to me that way. Usually it was "Ronald, come here and sit down." So I said, "What do you mean, lesson?"

"What's the lesson you've learned from this?"

"Well," I said, "I needed money to buy food."

The voice stopped me and said, "No, no, no. What did you need?"

"Well, I needed money—"

"No, no. What did you *need?*"

"Oh, I needed food."

"That's right. Cut out the middleman—you needed food. That's what I gave you."

As inexplicable as the idea to visit Sally had seemed, she was the answer to my prayer. When you pray for a job and you get an answer telling you to move to another state, or when you pray for a new relationship and you get an answer telling you to change your job, you may respond by saying, "No, I'm not doing that. I want a job, I don't want to move." Or, "No, I want a new relationship, I don't need a new job." In that case, your prayer can no longer be answered because what you are hearing is the path to the answer, but you don't want to hear it. Being alert to the form the answer may take is another aspect of congruency, which can perhaps be defined as "Thy will, not mine, be done."

If you remain congruent, you can avoid falling into the rut of praying in what I call negative energy. A prayer of negative energy might sound something like this: "God, I've got a difficulty (or a problem, or a challenge) and I need your help. I probably don't deserve it, but I am going to ask anyway." With this attitude, you feel deep down within your being that you probably deserve to be punished. You have been taught to pray that way, which amounts to "Here goes, and by God, what have I got to lose? It might come to pass."

To complicate matters further, sometimes the positive results of prayer do not look positive to us, as my encounter with Sally illustrates. When you pray, your programming or conditioning determines your belief—the beliefs of your parents, the beliefs of your government, the beliefs of your religious institution. How many of you have been programmed to believe that God is out to get you? Ask yourself what you really believe about God. As behavioral psychologist Shad Helmstetter describes it in his book *What to Say When You Talk to Yourself,*

It is our programming that sets up our beliefs, and the chain reaction begins.

1. Programming creates beliefs.

2. Beliefs create attitudes.

3. Attitudes create feelings.

4. Feelings determine actions.

5. Actions create results.

That's how the brain works.

If you believe that God is against you, that He's just sitting in heaven waiting for you to slip up so He can have His angels throw you into hell, then you are likely to misinterpret His response to your prayers.

There is one other important aspect of congruency to remember with respect to prayer. In the gospel of Mark, Jesus said, "Whatever you pray for, believe you have it and it will be yours." Then comes the big "but": when you pray, you must first forgive. When divine energy is making its way to you through prayer, it can't reach you until you provide a channel for it to move through you to others. Jesus is saying, as other enlightened masters have said and are still saying: If you want to move mountains, whatever those mountains of difficulty are, you must learn to forgive.

Making yourself a channel for divine energy is another way of stating the prayer of Saint Francis (see Appendix 1). One way I have defined prayer is as the exchange of light-energy between the human and the Divine. When you are truly in connection with God in prayer, and light-energy is moving between the human and the Divine, that power can sometimes become so strong it literally knocks people down. The reason that happens is that the human body is wired for only a certain amount of energy. When we make a very powerful connection with God, the energy of God begins to permeate us, and we begin to act like magnifying glasses. You know what happens when you focus a magnifying glass on paper or dry leaves so as to catch the rays of the sun and concentrate them. The sun's energy is always there, but by using the magnifying glass, you concentrate its power. When we pray, something very similar happens. For example, the healing services I do with large groups sometimes last three to four hours. Afterward my staff will say to me, "You must be exhausted." Unfortunately, just the opposite is usually the case; I become so energized that I cannot sleep. Often tremendous heat moves through me, and yet my body does not sweat and does not become weak or depleted; it actually becomes stronger. The only problem (apart from the insomnia) is that my hands and fingers often begin to blister.

This doesn't happen to everyone, nor should you look for it when you pray. Once you reach the higher level of prayer, you should have only one reason to pray—to be in communion with God. You want nothing more than God. If we are truly tuned in to God by prayer and meditation, then through what Saint Paul in his first letter to the Corinthians calls "the gifts of the Holy Spirit," and what in his letter to the Galatians he calls "the fruit of the Spirit," we become the eyes of God, the mind of God, the hands of God, the heart of God. Once you recognize that is your true essence, then you begin to be aware that you must see as God sees and think as God thinks. You must love as God loves and use your hands in a way that God would. That is divine congruency.

I've already discussed the ways in which God is light-energy. And since, as I have said repeatedly, we are made in the image of God, then we must have an energetic nature as well. To put this in modern physical terms, I would employ a phrase popularized by Dr. Herbert Benson in his book *Timeless Healing* and say that we are "wired for God." Anyone raised in the Jewish-Christian tradition knows the biblical quotation that says we are made "in the image and likeness of God." That line would probably be better rendered as "we are made in the image *as* the likeness of God." What's the distinction? To me, it's the difference between a noun and a verb. To think of myself as being made in God's image and likeness may be comforting: it means that I resemble the Creator in various ways. I'm a knockoff of God, like the five-dollar Rolex you can buy on any city street corner. But to think that I am made "*as* the likeness of God" means that I had better start acting like God *as an expression of His reality.* I can't sit back and admire His handiwork; I have to emulate Him, to be "as His likeness."

And so, along with maintaining awareness of God's response to us in prayer, if we are to be fully congruent with God we have to be aware of the attributes of God that are wired into our makeup. If our spiritual circuitry is the same as the spiritual circuitry of God, how is God wired?

God is love and compassion, and so we are wired for love and compassion. God is justice and mercy, and so we are wired for justice and mercy. God is faith, and so we are also wired for faith. If you don't believe that we are wired for faith, just think of the last time you prepared for a vacation by reciting a litany of all the things that would go wrong. The car would break down, the hotel would lose your reservation, the weather would be awful. When some of these things then occurred, instead of kicking the dog and yelling at your spouse, you should have exclaimed, "Hallelujah, Lord! Look at what my faith has produced!"

We have been wired by God for faith, but if we use that faith in a negative way, we will surely produce something negative. That's not God's fault. There's a marvelous story in the Old Testament about Moses leading the Israelites out of Egypt. When they come to the Red Sea, Moses begins to plead with God to do something. God says to Moses the same thing He so often says to me: "Shut up!" Then He instructs Moses to stretch forth his hand and divide the sea. In response, Moses has a classic "Aha!" experience. He realizes that he is wired with the power of God; trusting his spiritual intuition, he stretches forth his hand, divides the sea, and leads his people across.

The Jewish and Christian traditions being inextricably linked, we can easily find a parallel story in the New Testament. When Jesus is teaching in the countryside, the disciples tell him that the people are hungry and that Jesus should send them away to buy themselves something to eat. Jesus doesn't respond by saying, "I'll feed them." He says, "*You* give them something to eat." Read the text closely here. After Jesus blesses the five loaves, he gives them "to the disciples to set before the people" (Mark 6:37ff). The disciples perform the miracle themselves without even knowing it—because they are wired with that kind of power.

And so are all of us, if we only knew it. We have to begin to understand who we are. We are elegant spirits made in the image *as* the likeness of God. We are not God anymore than rays of sunshine are the sun, but we are emanations of God. That's why we are wired to excel, not to be mediocre. We are wired to be decisive. We are wired to be conquerors, because that's what God is—not in the sense of conquering other people but of conquering difficulty, of conquering ourselves. In Islam, there is a well-known hadith, or oral tradition, in which the Prophet Muhammad, returning from one of his battles against the enemies of the new religion, says to his followers, "We now turn from the lesser jihad to the greater jihad." The much misunderstood Arabic word "jihad" does not mean "holy war" but rather "struggle" or "exertion." For Muhammad, the "lesser jihad" meant the physical struggle against external adversaries; the more challenging struggle was the "greater jihad" against the selfish motives of our limited ego.

Every time we do something that is contrary to our spiritual circuitry, we are asking for trouble. The beauty of the spiritual life is that at any moment, if we can learn how to connect with God from the depths of our heart, we can open our channels to receive all the energy of God. At any moment, we can become the eyes and mind of God.

But to say that becoming the eyes and mind and hands and heart of God isn't easy is an understatement. Let's look, for instance, at how we are to become the mind of God. When we are plugged into prayer and are communicating on an authentic level with God, our barriers are down and we are letting God speak to us. We are letting ourselves be confronted by the presence of God about what needs to be enhanced or changed or healed in our lives. Many of us still believe that if we could only figure it out, things would become all right. But let me suggest that if you're approaching middle age and "figuring things out" hasn't worked up to this point, it's not going to work.

When we think about the mind of God and we look in Paul's first letter to the Corinthians, we find that we are wired for what is called the "word of knowledge," or the word of wisdom and spiritual understanding. Today we might call that clairaudience, clairvoyance, clairsentience—the moments in which you get revelations. You might be reading scripture, or you might have heard a priest or minister or rabbi preach on a particular passage. Maybe it never made sense to you before, but at this moment, all of a sudden your mind has opened up. Energy floods through you and you say, "My God, I know what this means to me." You have just tapped into the wisdom of God.

When you are looking for guidance, where do you go? How many counselors must you seek out before you finally sit back and say, "I think I'll talk to God about this"? Your wisdom channel may be clogged right now, but you are wired for that kind of wisdom if you would just open up to it. It's that simple. You are not entering into prayer or meditation for these reasons. You are there to become one with God, but in doing that you begin to open up your own channel and the wisdom begins to flow.

Congruency Applied: Finding Your Own Path

Although I have presented a number of exercises or techniques for prayer and healing in this book, I don't want to give the impression that these are the only ways to pray or seek guidance. I understand that techniques that work wonderfully for me may not always work as well for someone else. Besides, I doubt that most mystics found their paths in books, although they have often been inspired by reading the works of other mystics and then building upon them. So I hope that you, too, will be inspired to grow and discover your own unique ways of dealing with personal issues, to improvise your own strategies for spiritual unfolding, ones that are congruent with who you are.

Let me give you an example of one way I've found of dealing with psychological and emotional issues, in the hope that it may suggest or inspire something in you. Most of the times I've needed to ask God for guidance about an issue that was blocking me, I've been able to do so on a conscious level. Only on one or two occasions have I been "under the power" for five or ten minutes, meaning that as I prayed or as someone prayed for or with me I became unconscious and received an emotional or psychological healing on a deeper level. Usually I can just ask God to let me know what is blocking me or making me feel ill or upset. Then I go about my business, and I may receive an impulse later to go to the bookstore. As I'm walking down the aisle, a book will catch my attention and I'll pick it up. It may be dealing with self-esteem, for instance. That is the voice of God bringing the issue to the front and saying to me, "Here is what we need to work on. Now how are we going to work on this?"

Then I may be guided to take a passage from scripture and meditate on it. In this case, it could be that passage in the New Testament about the demoniac who ran among the tombs with no clothes on, crying out and bruising himself with stones (Mark 5:1–20). I may get a revelation that this man's problem was essentially one of self-esteem. I would then put myself in his place and see myself running around aimlessly. But I would also see myself kneeling before Jesus and asking him to help my self-esteem, and that would begin to yield results.

Now I invite you to set aside a prayer session to ask God's help with a particular personal issue that has been nagging at you and making you feel blocked. Ask for His guidance and remain open to whatever impulse or suggestion might come to you, either then or later in the day, or even at night in a dream. Follow up on the suggestions and bring the results back with you into your next prayer session. Continue to work with the issue in this way until you receive some insight into the problem. If you like, you may also use the following prayer from Psalm 139 to calm and clear your mind during these sessions:

> O Lord, you have searched me and you know me.
> You know when I sit and when I stand;
>   you perceive my thoughts from afar.
> You discern my going out and my lying down;
>   you are familiar with all my ways.
> Before a word is on my tongue
>   you know it completely, O Lord.

. . . .

Where can I go from your Holy Spirit?
For you created my inmost being;
  you knit me together in my mother's womb.
I praise you because I am wonderfully made;
  your works are wonderful, I know them full well.
My frame was not hidden from you
  when I was made in the secret place.
When I was woven together in the depths of the earth,
  your eyes saw my unformed body.
All the days ordained for me
  were written in your book
  before one of them came to be.

EVERYDAY
MYSTICISM

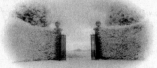

Apprehend God in all things, for God is in all things.
Every single creature is full of God and is a book about God.

◆

MEISTER ECKHART

No one spiritual concept causes more misunderstanding than "mysticism." The term can bring to mind wild-eyed fanatics and unbelievable accounts of psychic feats. Even those accomplishments that have been scientifically documented are often looked on with great skepticism, such as the ability of certain Asian holy men to lower their heart rate or respiration to astonishing levels or to dry sheets drenched in ice-cold water by raising their body temperature during meditation. What does mysticism have to do with being holy, anyway?

The word "mystic" derives from the same Greek root as does "mystery," a root meaning "close-mouthed," which was how members initiated into the Greek "mystery schools" were supposed to remain about what went on there. A sense of mystery has always shrouded mystical pursuits, but it is no longer necessary to be close-mouthed about the life of the spirit that mystics have traditionally explored.

I describe a mystic rather differently from the standard version. To me, a mystic is someone who has ascended the mount of transfiguration as Jesus did, and who has then returned to the flatland to become a center of creative energy and power in the world. In whatever life a mystic may engage, he or she partakes of the divine energy of God and becomes united with that ultimate Reality we call God in such a way that the world can no longer touch him or her. Hidden in God, inflamed with divine love, peacefully serene, the mystic possesses a creative strength and power that those of us caught up with our primitive self do not possess.

By this definition, I would consider myself a mystic-in-progress. I certainly wouldn't compare myself with Teresa of Ávila or Thérèse of Lisieux or Padre Pio or Yogananda, but I genuinely feel that's my calling—and yours, too. The reason I am writing this book is to help others avoid falling into the ruts I fell into. By sharing my own journey, I feel I can give others more hope to continue theirs.

Mysticism is not about the romantic withdrawing from the world into a monastery or ashram. It is not about entering into altered states of consciousness to experience blissful raptures variously known as *samadhi* or *satori* or the beatific vision. On the contrary, mysticism requires an understanding that true spirituality is about staying grounded. A spiritual person cuts the grass, makes dinner, does the dishes, and cleans the toilets. At one point in my spiritual practice, I mistakenly believed that everything should be done for me because I was devoting most of my time to prayer. The net result was that after a time, I felt burnt out. I didn't realize then that making dinner, doing the dishes, and cleaning the toilets can all be forms of prayer.

The seventeenth-century Christian mystic known as Brother Lawrence also talks about this everyday active prayer in a book called *The Practice of the Presence of God*. Formerly a footman and soldier by the name of Nicholas Herman of Lorraine, Brother Lawrence had a conversion experience at the age of eighteen that altered his life forever. While gazing at a winter tree stripped of all its leaves, he suddenly realized that it would shortly be renewed and would spring forth with flowers and fruit, and that the same was possible for him. Entering the monastery shortly afterward, he found joy in his daily work in the kitchen, which became a form of prayer for him. A correspondent of his wrote of Brother Lawrence, "that with him the set times of prayer were not different from other times; that he retired to pray, according to the directions of his superior, but that he did not want such retirement, nor ask for it, because his greatest business did not divert him from God."

Brother Lawrence knew that you cannot separate the spiritual life from the daily life of work and pleasure. I learned this lesson in a very distressing way in 1983, when still a parish priest approximately ninety miles from Chicago. As I was attempting to perform healing rituals and immerse myself in a life of prayer, I forgot that I was still in a human body. Endeavoring to focus on the "spiritual" side of life, I began to neglect the material altogether. I stopped doing the little pleasurable things that would have supplied balance in my life. I became depressed and disoriented. As somebody once put it, I was becoming so heavenly minded, I was no earthly good to anyone.

Many people are turned off to the spiritual life because they mistakenly believe that to be a mystic and live a holy life they will have to give up everything they love. Mysticism is not self-abnegation, however; it's living in harmony. To live a spiritual life you don't give up things, you bring joy and refreshment *into* your life. Psalm 16:11 declares, "O Lord, you've shown me the path to life; in your presence is fullness of joy, and in your right hand are pleasures forevermore." Of course, when Peter quotes that Psalm in the Book of Acts (2:25–28), he (or whoever wrote or later edited Acts) leaves off the last phrase about pleasures in the right hand of God. Somebody in the Church didn't think that the path of life, the fullness of joy, and pleasures belonged together.

In our own time, the Vietnamese Buddhist monk Thich Nhat Hanh teaches that living in the present moment, or mindfulness, is the aim of contemplation and meditation. The present moment includes everything, both spiritual and material. Thich Nhat Hanh teaches that we can be in a meditative state while walking the streets of a big, noisy city. You don't have to go to your room and sit in a lotus position for four hours to be meditative—unless, of course, you are guided to. Even if you are guided to solitary meditation, you can carry your deeply meditative state into your daily activities, like paying the bills or doing housework. We strive to be in the present moment because God is in the present.

We speak of the Divine Presence, but have you ever heard anyone refer to the Divine Future or the Divine Past? To live in the present moment means that you must be consciously aware and connected with the Source of all life in every moment of life—which is why taking prayer breaks throughout the day, for instance, is such an essential part of everyday mysticism. Being in the present moment also means letting go of regret for the past or fear of the future. If you have fears about death, about separation from your material existence or your loved ones, you will not be able to live in this present moment. Once we start plugging all of our circuits into the future or the past, we lose power rapidly because we forget how to live in the present. The purpose of prayer and meditation is to bring you back to where you belong in the present moment. To live this moment as fully as possible, right now, wherever you may be, is living in the presence of God. Zen Buddhists, who don't speak of God per se but who have made a science of living in the present, have a saying: "When eating, just eat; when walking, just walk." Be fully present in your simplest actions and do not overlay them with fantasies, fears, regrets, and other distractions.

Take a few minutes now as you are reading these words to perform one of the most familiar spiritual exercises of mystics from all the world's great traditions: being present. It is as simple as breathing and as difficult to maintain as keeping your balance on a tightrope—which is what the mystical author of the *Katha Upanishad* meant when he said that the spiritual path is as narrow and as difficult to follow as walking on the edge of a razor. (Jesus seems to be paraphrasing him in the Gospel of Matthew, 7:13: "For the gate is narrow and the way is hard, that leads to life, and those who find it are few.") We tend to fall to one side or the other of consciousness, either drifting into the past with nostalgic longing or regret, or sailing into the future with elaborate fantasies and plans of what we'll do tomorrow or next year. The aim of mystical life is to remain in the ever-changing present moment, rooted only in our awareness of the unchanging Divine.

Whether you are riding on a subway or an airplane, sitting at your desk or lying in bed, begin by taking note of every sound you can make out around you. Simply hear it, identify it in some way, and let it wash over and around you; then let it go. Notice the layers of distance, from the barely audible whir of a fan motor or ventilator or the chirping of birds just outside your window to the more distant sounds of an oil furnace in the basement, cars passing on the street below, sirens or tolling bells far off. Close your eyes if it helps.

Now carry on a similar process of observation for smells, including those that may be offensive, like chemical smells or the polluted odors of city air. Of course, don't ignore the many pleasant smells that may reach you from flowers or trees, the smells of food or perfume, or of your own body. Let each discrete smell enter your awareness, stay with it a moment, and then let it go, like a passing thought during meditation.

Now use your eyes to observe details of your physical environment. Take in colors, angles, designs abstract and geometrical, textures in the wood and metal and fabric and other components of whatever structure houses you. If you're fortunate enough to be outside, notice the materials that make up the buildings around you or, alternatively, the colors and textures of the trees and grass and rock outcroppings of the natural world. Let your vision extend as far as possible, even if it is only to the corner of the ceiling in your bedroom, where a cobweb wavers in the updraft from a heating unit. Notice with equanimity both the beauty of certain objects and designs and the flaws and imperfections in them.

If there are any people around you, take note of them. Or, if you are alone in a room, extend your awareness in concentric layers to other rooms of your house or apartment, the next house over or the apartments surrounding you, the roads and buildings beyond. Be aware that these other people are inhabiting the same world, breathing the same air, suffering the same sorrows and aspiring to the same joys as you are. In effect, they are connected to you, however tenuous or even irritating the threads may seem that bind you together. Feel love for them at least on some level, and let that love be a reflection of the love you feel for yourself.

Finally, be aware of your own body, emotions, and mind. Be alert to any physical sensations you may feel as you conduct this exercise, any feelings of heat or cold, comfort or irritation, and notice from which part of your body they emanate. Gently direct loving attention to that part of your body where you feel pain, tension, or discomfort. Without judging your body for these sensations, allow the light of the Holy Spirit to engulf them. Be aware that, with a few exceptions, we generally exist in what one modern mystic terms "an ocean of bliss." We may not be aware of the good feelings that are constantly circulating within our bodies until we allow ourselves to be still and experience them. But whatever arises is part of what you are at this moment in your journey; honor each sensation for what it is, and then release it.

Observe your emotional state during the exercise. Is it swept by feelings of impatience, awkwardness, frustration, comfort, peace, or bliss? Genuine meditation may also evoke deeper feelings and memories, as often unpleasant and troubling as fanciful or delightful. Without judging or trying to evaluate these feelings, simply look to see if there is anything you can learn about yourself from their presence. Honor them, and then let go of them. Don't let your emotions carry you off into fantasies of guilt or shame or self-aggrandizement; always bring yourself gently back to the present moment.

The mind can be especially troublesome during prolonged or

even brief periods of sitting meditation and prayer. According to the classic Indian simile, the mind is like a monkey, leaping aimlessly from branch to branch, taking you with it as you attempt to follow each new thought or fantasy. It may take some time to come to terms with this "monkey mind," as it is called. Most of us never learn to completely control it, but that isn't absolutely necessary now. At least learn to watch its vagaries, see how it takes you from concentration on the Divine to endless ruminations about what your spouse or lover said to you this morning, what you'll be having for dinner, or how you'll meet all your expenses. Watch your mind doing this, remind yourself what's happening, and gently call it back to focus. That's one reason sacred images are useful tools for meditation; they give your mind something to focus on each time it wanders off into the jungle. Returning your attention to your breath is also an effective technique when the mind wanders; no judgment is implied, simply a remembrance that the breath represents the action of the Holy Spirit, the Breath of God, within you.

Through this process, become aware of yourself not as an isolated individual but as someone intimately connected to the world—not only to other beings but also to the sounds and smells and sights that surround you. These are all expressions of God's light-energy, no matter how dim or distantly remembered. Although we should aim to see ourselves as spirit traveling temporarily in a body, we should never denigrate that body, or matter in general, because it, too, comes from God. Above all, we aim to balance our awareness of the body, the mind, the emotions, and our overarching spiritual consciousness, leaving out none of these areas. To focus only on the spiritual realm and to attempt to ignore the physical, for instance, can lead to feelings of being "spaced out" or ungrounded. This realization is at the heart of what it means to be "in the world but not of the world."

You can repeat this practice virtually anytime, anywhere.

Mystics often use it as a prelude to prayer and meditation, but like many an appetizer, if prepared lovingly it can sometimes serve as a main course. Being in the present moment in this way may also help to dispel some of our residual disdain for the everyday world. Maybe the problem is not that we are too absorbed in the material world but that we are often lost in our own fantasies about it, dreaming about the past or scheming for the future, floating disconnected from both the Creator and creation—not really *in* the world at all. By learning to be fully present, we can anchor ourselves spiritually as well as physically. This is the heart and soul of everyday mysticism, and can perhaps be thought of as a prerequisite for prayer. At the very least, it is a solid foundation on which to build a substantial and enduring prayer life.

In *The Interior Castle,* Saint Teresa of Ávila took the scriptural quotation of Jesus' "In my Father's house are many mansions" and picked out seven rooms to show the ascent into the highest form of prayer. She goes from the "gimme" prayers to divine union, in which you seek nothing but God. In *The Ascent of Mount Carmel,* John of the Cross talks about ten levels of prayer. The numbers are not important, unless you want to compare them with the Vedic system of seven chakras or the Kabbalistic Tree of Life with its ten *sefirot.* What is important is that you always have an opportunity to ascend. God is always offering us a choice of whether to stay where we are or to move on. Mystics, knowing this, will never attack another's religion or spiritual path, because they know we always have a choice. They know that, as the famous line from the Rig Veda puts it, "Truth is one, but sages call it by different names." A true mystic understands that God is all-inclusive.

In the last line of Chapter 5 from the Gospel of Matthew, Jesus tells his disciples to "be perfect, even as your heavenly Father is perfect." This is the kind of oft-quoted scripture that makes you want to throw up your hands and say, "What's the use? I'll never be perfect!" Yet the line has been wrongly translated and taken out of context. The original meaning of the word translated as "perfect" is "complete," "all-embracing," or "all-inclusive": "to be all-inclusive as God is all-inclusive." Inclusiveness *is* a kind of perfection, but the two terms are hardly interchangeable. In the context of the quote, Jesus has just been saying that we must love not only our neighbors but also our enemies, because the Father in heaven "makes his sun rise on the evil and on the good, and sends rain on the just and on the unjust." Jesus is clearly talking about inclusiveness in a sense that would be recognized by any Vedantic, Taoist, or Buddhist mystic. His intent is to let us know that we are wired for love, and that love includes everybody; it makes no distinction between Catholics and Protestants, or Jews or Muslims or Hindus or atheists.

Contrary to the romantic image of the spacey, otherworldly spiritual person, mystics are extremely practical. Saint Teresa, one of the greatest mystics of the medieval church, could be quite reasonable. When one of the nuns in her province complained that she couldn't get along with one of the other sisters, Teresa replied, "The next time you see her walking down the hall, walk on the other side." On another occasion, Teresa was going to visit one of her convents in a driving rainstorm. The driver hit a rut and Teresa was thrown from the carriage, landing facedown in the mud. Fortunately, she was unharmed, but as she lifted herself out of the mud she clenched her fist at the heavens and said, "Lord, if this is the way you treat your friends, no wonder you have so few!"

One good reason for seeing mysticism or spirituality as practical is that this perspective prevents you from saying, as many Christians do, "I'm saved," or, "I'm just waiting for the Rapture." I always ask them, "Saved from what?" I haven't yet received an adequate answer. The irony of the Rapture is that, despite the fact that fundamentalist Christianity is supposed to teach a return to the original doctrine of Jesus, that doctrine emerged only in the early twentieth century, based on a questionable reading of a verse from 1 Thessalonians (4:17).

You don't need dogma or doctrine to experience God. Very few canonized saints of the Catholic Church were drawn from the ranks of bishops and popes—and I can understand why. A surprising percentage of saints were simple folk, like Saint Francis of Assisi or Saint Clare, who didn't have degrees and never formally studied the doctrine of the Church. Even the Church itself has been forced to recognize this. Although Francis was never even ordained, the order of Franciscans he founded became one of the most influential orders of Catholic religious in the world.

Nonetheless, so much delicious truth still resides in some of the old rituals of the Church that they are worth reviving, if we can recover the original sense of what they mean. In the past, for instance, when the Gospel was read aloud, the priest and the people together would make the sign of the cross with their thumb and forefinger on the forehead, lips, and heart as they said, "Christ be on my mind, Christ be on my lips, Christ be in my heart." That prayer had a direct relationship to the desire to open the upper chakras to be transformed by the power of the sacred writings.

The system of chakras—centers of subtle energy or consciousness corresponding to seven areas of the physical body from the tailbone to the crown of the head—was developed in the East and has long been known to Hindus, Buddhists, and Taoists. The chakras have been variously interpreted by modern Western practitioners as well, but they are generally understood to represent a progression from our most instinctual, survival-oriented energies at the base of the spine upward to our most spiritual aspirations.

Although the system was not openly studied in Western religion, its centers were known intuitively by the mystics who entered into deep states of meditation. It is no coincidence that the sign of the cross was made on locations corresponding to the higher chakras: the fourth, or heart chakra, which represents love and compassion; the fifth chakra, centered behind the throat and related to personal expression and creativity; and the sixth chakra, known in the Western esoteric system as the third eye, which is regarded as the seat of consciousness. Likewise, the Tibetan Buddhist (Vajrayana) system speaks of the three centers of Body, Speech, and Mind, which correspond roughly to the heart, throat, and forehead.

In the old Christian tradition, making the sign of the cross on the heart, forehead, and lips was meant to open the heart to the Word, to align the will, and to live it in daily life. This kind of mystical knowledge was also embedded in many of the Church's rituals, although the understanding behind them was not always transmitted or retained. We have forgotten what many of the Church's oldest rituals were intended to accomplish and where they were supposed to direct our attention. Yet their potential to help us if we maintain the right attention and intention is great.

In the chapter that follows, I will offer ways to revive what I believe to be the original mystical intent behind the rituals known as the Seven Sacraments. First, however, I would like to take a brief look at one of the oldest and simplest rituals in the Christian tradition.

In mystical Christianity, clearly the greatest symbol of power was the cross, but the early Christian mystics understood it quite differently from people today. To the mystics, the cross was symbolic of spiritual energy. The vertical bar was the Light of God coming from heaven and interpenetrating Form. Where it penetrated, the Light expanded outward to all that was around it. At its center, it focused and concentrated the divine energy in much the same way that a powerful lens concentrates sunlight into fire. In old paintings or icons of saints and mystics, the figures are often depicted with their hands across their laps, or Jesus is shown holding down the last two fingers with his thumb while the index and middle finger point upward. Jesus isn't just showing us a neat way to pray; the saints and Jesus are physically completing the circle of energy, the spiritual circuitry.

The Kabbalah in Jewish mysticism embodies much the same concept. When Christians make the sign of the cross, they may say, "In the name of the Father, and of the Son, and of the Holy Spirit. Amen." Or they may say, "For thine is the kingdom, and the power, and the glory, now and forever. Amen." The Kabbalist also makes the sign of the cross, using Kabbalistic terms from the Hebrew that parallel Christian terminology. In *The New Living Qabalah*, Kabbalistic scholar Will Parfitt describes the cross as a healing tool for aligning one's energy and serving as a barrier against unwanted energetic intrusions. Because I feel that he has rediscovered much of the mystical power in the sign of the cross that Christians have forgotten, I will close this chapter with an exercise taken from his work.

THE KABBALISTIC CROSS

Parfitt recommends familiarizing yourself with this procedure and then practicing it at least daily, until it becomes second nature. You may then use it to begin any of the meditations, rituals, or mystical practices in this book, especially the exercise of being present included earlier in this chapter. Be sure to read the chart of pronunciations and meanings of the Hebrew terms at the end before beginning the exercise.

Stand upright, attentive but not stiff.

Touch your forehead (midway between and slightly above the eyebrows) with the forefinger of your right hand. Say:

ATEH

Be aware of the innermost self residing within you.

Move your finger down in a straight line to touch your genital area. Say:

MALKUTH

Be aware of your body.

Visualize this straight line down the front of your body, and all the subsequent lines you draw as bright, shining, silver-white light.

Touch your right shoulder. Say:

VE GEBURAH

Be aware of your will power.

Drawing a line across from your right shoulder, touch your left shoulder. Say:

VE GEDULAH

Be aware of your love energy. (Gedulah is another name for Chesed.)

Clasp your two hands together over your heart. Visualize a shining white cross inscribed over your body. Say:

LE OLAHM

Be aware of exactly where you are (here), exactly at this moment (now).

Extend your arms out so you are standing as a cross, and say:

AMEN

Visualize yourself extending as a silver-white cross in each of the four directions (up, down, right, left).

	PRONOUNCED	MEANS
ATEH	"AHTEH"	"FOR THINE"
MALKUTH	"MALKUT"	(IS THE) "KINGDOM"
VE GEBURAH	"VER GEBOORAH"	"THE POWER"
VE GEDULAH	"VER GEDOOLAH"	"THE GLORY"
LE OLAHM	"LE OHLARM"	"FOR EVER AND EVER"

Pronounce each word very slowly, and really stretch the vowels. The more energy you put into intoning the words, and the more will and imagination you use whilst doing this, the more effective it will be.

Don't rush it—be clear with each stage before you move on to the next. The inner meaning of the procedure is much more important than the outer form.

NEW SACRAMENTS
AS DAILY RITUALS

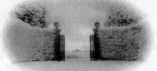

And you shall be to me a kingdom of priests and a holy nation.

◆

EXODUS 19:6

The old Baltimore Catechism of the Roman Catholic Church defined a sacrament as "an outward sign instituted by Christ to give grace." That was later expanded in the new *Catechism of the Catholic Church,* although the meaning remains essentially the same: "The sacraments are efficacious signs of grace, instituted by Christ and entrusted to the Church, by which divine life is dispensed to us." Aside from the part about their being entrusted to the Church, I could probably go along with most of that description, especially if by "divine life" we understand divine *energy.* But my own definition would be simpler than that. To me, a sacrament is a sacred ritual that acts as a vehicle for divine energy to be released for some specific purpose.

Sacraments can take the form of a sacred blessing or a time of prayer and communion with God, in which the participants may experience God tangibly either by themselves or in the context of a community of believers. These rituals are not to be considered rigid, empty formulas but vehicles for the life-giving energy that results from the connection between the human and the Divine that is at the heart of all authentic prayer. Yet we must be aware of what is happening in these moments to be able to experience a definite presence that heals and restores. As that presence emits energy, we receive the energy and allow it to do its healing work. The name we give these ritual events, whether baptism, confirmation, communion, or matrimony, is irrelevant. All that matters is what the event ought to bring about in us and through us.

In the course of my years as a spiritual healer, I have seen people healed at these ritual gatherings by being aware of energy moving about in one form or another. On several occasions, I have observed supernatural phenomena during confirmation and communion services. One that stands out most powerfully in my mind took place a few years ago during a communion service for healing in northern California. During this service, a woman who had been suffering from throat cancer came up to receive the communion elements (bread and wine). The cancer was so advanced that she was not sure she would be able to take communion at all. She had actually come to the service that night to pray for a friend of hers who had also been diagnosed with cancer.

Coming forward for communion, she took a particle of the bread in her mouth and did her best to swallow it. When she returned home later, her throat began to open up. She soon discovered that she was able to drink and eat for the first time in weeks without the tremendous pain that had previously shot through her throat. Within two days of taking communion, she went back to her doctor, who pronounced her completely cured of the cancer.

Although I had performed that communion service according to the book, I do not accept the notion that sacramental rituals must be strictly adhered to for their effects to be felt. Faith in a doctrine or dogma is not required to produce results, either. Very few if any healings occur with this kind of belief. Healings can occur, however, when we maintain an awareness of God's love for everyone and when we trust in His willingness to allow Himself to be experienced, even through what we interpret as supernatural phenomena. It is essential that we take advantage of the energy available to us in these rituals by participating in them even without the aid of clergy. As God's children, we have permission to enter into His presence on our own, whether at home or in any other environment. This idea is even supported by the theological belief that when Jesus died at the crucifixion and the veil of the Temple was ripped from the top to the bottom, God was saying that the Holy of Holies was no longer off-limits to the laity. Through the death of Jesus, the gates were swung wide open for anyone to enter.

Since I feel that the original significance of the sacraments has been obscured if not entirely lost over the centuries, I would like to propose a new understanding of each of them. I also believe that sacraments such as baptism, confirmation, and ordination, which were customarily performed only once in life, can in fact be used on a regular basis to release in each of us the divine energy associated with them.

Several of the following rituals call for blessed water or oil. You can obtain blessed water from most Catholic, Orthodox, or Episcopal churches by calling the parish and asking for it; many churches keep large containers of holy water in the lobby. I make my own blessed oil by combining any high-quality olive oil with some fragrant oils such as cinnamon, frankincense, and myrrh (which you can find in the aromatherapy section of many health food stores) and saying a short blessing over it. Simply ask the Holy Spirit to infuse the oil with the power and presence of God in this fashion: "Come, Holy Spirit, breathe your life force into this object, oil, so that every person anointed with this oil will experience your healing touch on some level of their being. Amen."

Ordination

Normally, the list of sacraments begins with baptism. But because the current Catholic conception of the sacraments presupposes a priestly class of celibate men endowed with the sole power to administer them, I would rather begin with the sacrament of Holy Orders, which I prefer to call ordination. To get away from the belief that we need a clerical class to intervene on our behalf, I propose a new definition of ordination as the blessing of what we are called by God to do and to be. We are each called to do a specific work according to our talents, abilities, and personality, and that amounts to a new sense of priesthood. In keeping with our role as everyday mystics, this priesthood represents how we are to be a channel for God in the secular, workaday world as opposed to living solely in the monastery, ashram, cloister, or temple. As God told Abraham, a priest is someone who is blessed in order to be a blessing to others.

If we are each to act as our own priest as I am suggesting, we need to understand how to bless our work on a daily basis. The last verse of Psalm 90 in the Amplified Version of the Bible reads: "And let the beauty and delightfulness and favor of the Lord our God be upon us; confirm and establish the work of our hands, yes, the work of our hands confirm and establish it."

The psalmist in essence is asking the Lord to bless his daily work—"the work of our hands." And that's what I would like to enable each of you to do on your own, in the same vein in which the Lord instructed Moses on Mount Sinai to tell the people of Israel that they were to be a nation of priests. I recommend that this ritual be performed at the beginning of the work week, perhaps on a Sunday evening or Monday morning. Whenever I leave to go to a conference or workshop, for instance, I take some holy water and bless all the books and tapes that my associate, Paul Funfsinn, will be selling there—not so much for any monetary return but so they will be a blessing on the lives of the people who buy and use them. Whether you are a shoe salesman or a plumber, a homemaker or an artist or a corporate lawyer, you can use this five-minute ritual to bless your own work for the day. Take some blessed water and sprinkle it over the tools of your work, whatever they might be. Then recite the words from Psalm 90 that I just quoted, and dedicate your work to God. You may also say this prayer:

"Lord God, I ask you to bless this work that will fulfill and heal not only my life but also the lives of thousands of others who will be affected by this work. I ask you now to establish the work of my hands, the work that you have called me to do. Let it be a blessing now not only to me but to others. Amen."

Placing a blessing on our work further makes us aware that our calling is a sacred one, and that awareness makes us more apt to be genuinely oriented toward the service of others. If you think of your work as sacred, you will be less likely to want to cheat someone, do shoddy work, or do work that harms others—a principle the Buddha referred to as "right livelihood." The money that comes from our work, then, is not an end in itself but the means to an end in that it gives us the freedom to be priests in our own right.

Baptism

In the Book of Genesis, God creates water and everything else after He creates light (energy). Throughout biblical imagery, water is conceived as the great carrier or conductor of God's essence: in the waters of the flood, the parting of the Red Sea, or the waters of the Jordan where John baptized. Baptism could become a more powerful tool for healing if churches would abandon or at least lessen their emphasis on the archaic concepts of original sin and regeneration and focus on the energizing effects of water.

The water of baptism calls us to immerse our whole being in the energy of God, which is love, resulting in a rebirth and renewal that is more plausible than being baptized for the "forgiveness of sins." In baptism we have the chance to return consciously to our original state as spirit and to see ourselves as cocreators with God, having the power and ability to reestablish the earth as a Garden of Eden.

In the Christian concept, baptism was intended to signify our symbolic entrance into the family of God, making us children of the Lord. But since I believe that we are born as emanations of God, we do not need to be formally inducted into His family. In a daily, practical manner, however, we can use baptism and the other sacraments to provide us with the sacred energy to perform whatever tasks we face. Water is used in baptism because it has always been associated by every major religion on earth with life, with cleansing and revivification. This is not merely symbolic; a real energy is released by our contact with water, which is why we feel so invigorated and relaxed after taking a shower or bath. Yet if you recognize the sacred value of water, you can feel yourself immersed in the life of God.

In Genesis, the Holy Spirit or Holy Breath of God was brooding (waiting to create) over the void (emptiness). When God spoke, the Spirit was activated and began to create. When God spoke and breathed, healing and creative properties, the reconstructive energy in the Breath of God, brought something into existence out of apparent nothingness. As children of God's light, we are on this planet to continue the work of creation. (It may not be completely accurate, however, to speak of bringing creation into existence out of nothing. In his book *Learning to Dance Inside*, George Fowler eloquently makes the following distinction: "The Judeo-Christian creation myth in the Bible, essentially matching the many creation tales of other cultures, tells of a divine artisan making all things out of nothing. . . . But . . . eternal Being didn't reach into nothingness and create things. It simply outpressed expression of Its own existence from the field of infinite possibility that Being by Its very nature is.")

Unlike the Old Testament, the New Testament defines no need for a mediator. We're it! Jesus did away with the role of mediator by returning to the original plan of God for the Israelites to be a nation of priestly people. They, like us, by virtue of being God's children, were to have direct access to God if they accepted their role as priests. In large measure, they didn't. For that reason, I believe, God allowed the concept of a separate priesthood to be established, although this produced dire consequences and, in Christianity today, still does. Now we have an opportunity for what the Jews call *tikkun*—restoration.

Returning to the ritual of baptism through which we are made aware of our nature as spirit, we symbolically begin our journey of unfolding consciousness. As I have stated, the early Christian Church brought new converts "into the fold" through the initiation rites of baptism, confirmation, and communion, each ritual granting a grace (empowerment) for the purpose of one's spiritual unfoldment. These three sacraments were spiritual channels for healing. In fact, the ritual of confirmation was often accompanied by speaking in tongues, healing, prophecy, resting in the spirit, and experiencing divine electrical energy in one form or another. The early Christians understood that these events ought to occur as stated by Saint Paul in Chapter 12 of his first letter to the Corinthian Church, "concerning spiritual gifts." This, however, no longer appears to be the case. Grace in the form of energy that produces supernatural phenomena is neither expected nor desired on the part of the hierarchy of most Christian churches. And so, in a literal sense, we have to take matters into our own hands.

To baptize yourself, I suggest you fill a bathtub with water and put some blessed water in it. In the old Christian Easter ritual, which is no longer a part of the Catholic tradition, the priest would bend over the water and breathe upon it, recognizing that the Breath of God—the Source of all life—was flowing through him. We can reclaim that tradition by breathing on the bathwater while repeating the words of the sign of the cross ("In the name of the Father, and of the Son, and of the Holy Spirit"). If you feel uncomfortable with that prayer, you can simply say, "I breathe upon you the life of God," or any words that come to you intuitively in that situation.

Before getting into the bathtub, say the following prayer or, if you have a battery-powered tape recorder, you can prerecord the prayer and play it back.

"Father-Mother, divine Parent, you give us grace through sacred signs and symbols that tell us of the wonders of your unseen energy. In baptism we use your gift of water, which you have made a rich symbol of the grace you give us in this sacramental sign. At the very dawn of creation, your Spirit breathed on the waters, making them the wellspring of your divine energy. The waters of the great Flood you made a sign of the waters of cleansing that bring an end to the past and make a new beginning of goodness in the present moment. Through the waters of the Red Sea, you led Israel out of slavery to be an image of God's holy people, a nation of priests set free from all past bondages through your divine healing, cleansing love, symbolized by the baptismal waters. In the waters of the Jordan, Jesus was baptized by John and anointed with the Holy Spirit, reminding us of our inheritance as God's children, heirs to all that is good. After his Resurrection, Jesus told his disciples to go out and teach all nations, immersing them in the energizing life of the Father and of the Son and of the Holy Spirit.

"Lord, look now with love upon me and unseal for me the energy of baptism. By the power of the Holy Spirit, please give to me now the grace of healing and transformation. You created me in your own likeness; cleanse me from all darkness that hinders my healing and transformation."

Now light a candle and briefly hold its base in the tub as a sign of God's spiritual energy penetrating the form we call water. You may say as you do so, "Springs of water, bless the Lord. Give Him glory and praise forever." Then, with conscious awareness, immerse your body slowly in the water. Become aware that an energy is passing through the water and into you, not only physically but also on a spiritual level. Soak up the spiritual energy that has passed into the water from the act of blessing it and mingling it with blessed water.

Reconciliation (Confession)

The tradition of the self-examination or daily review extends back to the earliest days of Christian mysticism. The focus of the sacrament of Penance, as it became known in the Catholic Church, shifted away from examination to acknowledging one's guilt and paying a penalty. But self-examination is not the same as self-flagellation, and can be performed without blame or regret. The only one who needs to know your dark side is you. The sacrament of confession or reconciliation isn't so much between another person and myself as it is between my lower self and my higher self. When I reconcile my inner selves, I am able to be more loving and accepting of others, and healing can take place—both spiritual and physical.

One of the best times I know for practicing confession is during the baptismal bath. You might want to invoke the Holy Spirit and then call to mind the actions of the day, both those that were a blessing to others and those that may literally have been curses to others. You may recall times when you weren't being the best instrument of God's peace that you could have been, even if you had no direct contact with the person involved, such as when you mentally curse someone for cutting you off in traffic.

Allow the presence of the Holy Spirit to surround you as you review the events of the day and your part in them without blame, judgment, condemnation, resentment, or bitterness. When you recall some event in which you feel you acted as a channel of God's peace, ask the Holy Spirit to expand that further into your life. When the Spirit brings to your mind those moments in which you embodied less than the Christ nature, ask the Lord to forgive you and to help you replace those actions with greater love and greater awareness of kindness. You don't need to engage in elaborate analysis of your actions and motivations. The image that comes to mind here is of stirring up the bottom of a pond and watching the debris come to the surface. As you observe, if you see junk that you don't want to be there, let it rise to the surface of your consciousness so the Holy Spirit can dissolve it with light. If you have a battery-operated tape recorder, you can play chants from any sacred tradition. Sacred chants have a vibrational frequency that can touch the core of our being, and by their gentle resonance they can begin to shake loose the negative barnacles that may have accumulated on the spiritual level of our being.

Of course, you don't need to take a bath to have confession. You can easily do a self-examination in the last ten minutes before you fall asleep at night. It may be easier to make this a daily habit if you aren't disposed to taking long baths at night. As you lie in your bed with the lights out, perform the examination I just described. You may even find this ritual will help relieve your mind of troubled thoughts arising from the day's activities and ease your transition to the sleep state. Because of this sacrament's ability to put your heart at ease, there is no need to conclude it with a special prayer. Simply allow your heart to be filled with gratitude at God's mercy as you drift off to sleep.

Confirmation

We came into this life as emanations of God's light, fire, spark, spirit, yet our minds often become so clouded by the cares and anxieties of life that we forget we are spirit. So we need to take some time in solitude to remind ourselves that the Spirit of the Lord God is alive within us, and that the Spirit is our strength. Our need for solitude is the principle behind the sacraments of baptism and confession as I've conceived them. In solitude we recall that the true self is not weak; on the contrary, the eternal I AM presence of God within us is strong.

This is also the value of the sacrament of confirmation. The Latin roots of the word "confirmation" imply a desire to make firm the strength of God within us, confirming that in our very weakness we are strong. Saint Paul writes that the Lord said to him, "My grace is sufficient for you, for my power is made perfect in weakness" (2 Cor. 12:9). And the prophet Zephaniah said, "The Lord thy God in the midst of thee is mighty" (Zeph. 3:17). Before performing a healing ritual, I would often meditate on that verse and it would relax me so that I could allow the I AM Spirit to move through me and touch and heal people. That is true confirmation.

The grace of empowerment in the ritual of confirmation strengthens our awareness of God's Spirit dwelling in us, filling the universe with the divine energy of God's presence. This is what can be expected when one is "confirmed," no matter what one's "religious" beliefs are. The veil of unawareness is removed from the spiritual eye and one literally "sees the light." What a sense of strength comes from this new awareness, enabling us to proceed on our journey of spiritual unfoldment.

The ritual for confirmation can begin by lighting a candle, taking three deep breaths, and looking deeply at the flame of the candle. The flame signifies that the almighty presence of God's love is within you. Then take some blessed oil and place it on your forehead as a sign of the presence of the Holy Spirit within you (either daubing it or making the sign of the cross with your thumb), strengthening you for the activities of that day. You may also say, "I am strengthened by the awareness of God's almighty love burning within me."

Anointing the Sick

This sacrament used to be called Extreme Unction or the Last Rites, but those names represent a misunderstanding of its true benefit. For one thing, it is a healing sacrament that is properly applied to anyone who is sick. However, the same ritual can be performed for yourself, in which case you can make these blessings on your own body. Nowhere in the Bible does it say that you can't lay hands on yourself!

The person you are anointing, whether it's yourself or another, does not need to be bedridden by any means, but lying down for the administering of this sacrament symbolizes the desire to surrender to a more powerful force. The person may lie on a bed or couch for ten minutes as you invoke the prayer to the Holy Spirit ("Come, Holy Spirit") that appears in the following chapter. You can have the prayer on a tape recorder or let a third party read it aloud to leave your hands and mind free for the rest of the ritual. As you hear the words being said, put a little blessed oil on your thumb and make the sign of the cross on that part of the body where the illness is centered. (If that is not convenient or comfortable, simply make the sign of the cross on the forehead or heart.) Think of your personal understanding of the sign of the cross, and think also of the Kabbalistic concept of the cross as the light energy of God moving and penetrating every aspect of matter, infusing it with grace or sacred energy. Try to be aware of all these levels in some way as you make the sign, even if you do not verbalize them mentally.

The aim of the sacrament of anointing the sick is to open the higher energy centers to God's healing energy so that, if possible, person may be healed. As Dr. Larry Dossey has pointed out, the best resolution of an illness is not necessarily always a healing; sometimes the best resolution is that the person will die. But anointing the sick should at a minimum render the individual open to the healing energy of God, and should never be thought of merely as "last rites" for the dying.

Communion

Therese Neumann, the German Catholic stigmatist who was a contemporary of Padre Pio, completely abstained from food and drink for thirty years, except for the daily consumption of a communion wafer, yet remained the same weight throughout her life. In 1935, the Hindu mystic Paramahansa Yogananda, who showed a greater understanding of Christian scripture than most Western theologians, went to Germany to visit Therese and came away convinced of her authenticity, an encounter that he recorded in his classic work, *Autobiography of a Yogi*. When Yogananda, no stranger to seemingly impossible yogic feats, asked Therese how she was able to survive without eating, she replied through an interpreter, "I live by God's light."

"I see you realize that energy flows to your body from the ether, sun, and air," Yogananda responded. "Your sacred life is a daily demonstration of the truth uttered by Christ: 'Man shall not live by bread alone, but by every word that proceedeth out of the mouth of God.'"

Therese was delighted to be so readily understood by a fellow mystic, despite their surface differences in language, culture, and spiritual practice. "It is indeed so," she told him. "One of the reasons I am here on earth today is to prove that man can live by God's invisible light, and not by food only."

Yet food and communal dining are so much a part of human culture that Jesus sanctified both during his celebration of the Passover seder that has become known as the Last Supper. That sanctification is embodied in the sacrament of holy communion, a sacred ritual meant to remind us of our commonality with the Creator and with all creation. Communal meals have traditionally been the time when most cultures could express feelings of commonality. In many Eastern cultures, for instance, even during the most warlike times, sharing a meal with another precluded committing violence against him. The blood sacrifices of the Aztecs, Vedic Hindus, Israelites, and many others, which often included sharing the sacrificed animal, can be seen as early forms of a sacred communal meal.

You might consider having your communion service on Sunday morning as a way of starting the calendar week. Take a piece of bread and a little wine or grape juice in a glass. If you are Christian and are comfortable with the words, you could say, "This is my body" and "This is my blood" while consuming the bread and wine. But keep in mind that you are also saying that of yourself: "This is my life that I share with others." Just as God gave us His life, we give ours in service to others. This is a time to express gratitude for who you are and what life is about. In fact, gratitude is the most important element of a true communion service; the Greek word from which we get "Eucharist," or communion, means literally "a giving of thanks."

Although it isn't necessary to have others present, this sacrament does release an energy for bonding and partnership. It may be an especially valuable ritual for spouses or life partners or for a small gathering of like-minded people. The early Christians often gathered to share a meal and talk about the blessings in their lives. At one moment during the gathering, they would lift up the bread and wine and reiterate the words of Jesus before continuing the celebration of the meal. That one sacred moment pointed them toward God in the communal setting.

In a larger sense, a communal service like this can help us remember to be aware of the presence of God in the world, and how, as Therese Neumann pointed out, God's energy flows into us continually. As we become more consciously aware of those times when we have experienced the God presence, we may begin to realize the deep truth in the words of Jesus that "where two or more are gathered together in my name, there am I in the midst of them" (Matt. 18:20). The practical side of this awareness is that whenever people gather to break bread and lift a cup together, a presence is among them. Even business luncheons or meals at conference seminars can be times to enhance our experience of communal joy.

After consuming the food and drink, you may say this prayer:

Divine Parent, Creator of the cosmos, Source of all life, we do well always and everywhere to give you thanks. At the Last Supper, as Jesus sat at table with his Apostles, he offered himself to you as a Son, an acceptable gift that gives you praise. Jesus has given us this sacred communion meal to bring us its healing energy until the end of time. In this meal, Lord God, you feed your people and you strengthen them, so that the family of humankind may come to walk in the light of trust and confidence in one communion of love. We come then to be fed at your table and to grow into the likeness of the Christed One. Earth unites with heaven to sing a new song of creation as we adore and praise you forever. Amen.

Marriage

Saint Paul reminds us that marriage between man and woman symbolizes the mystical union between Christ and his church or

God and His people. This physical union, however, also symbolizes a much deeper union that is necessary before anyone can experience the beauty of honest relationships, even if one is still single. On a symbolic level, the ritual of marriage offers us the opportunity to embrace ourselves fully by uniting our shadow side with the part of us that we are able to accept openly. This union integrates both sides of us, allowing us to be in harmony with our total nature. A tremendous power is released by the integration of our total selves.

On yet another level, we can view the sacrament of marriage from the standpoint of the sacred energy emitted through a ritual of holy partnership. That partnership occurs first with God, then with oneself, and third with all creation. The purpose of this ritual is to make the participants aware that they are in partnership for healing the planet and bringing the light of God to the awareness of others.

To begin the ritual, light three candles to represent the three aspects of partnership—God, oneself, and all creation. Next, light some incense, both to symbolize your prayer rising to God and to remind you that you are a sweet perfume to God the Creator, the Source of all life. Then you may read from a sacred scripture dealing with partnership or cocreation. Pick one of your own or choose from the following texts, which derive from a number of different religious traditions and all of which come from the anthology *World Scripture,* compiled by Andrew Wilson. Although these scriptures and others you may choose refer to husband and wife and children, you may interpret them as follows: The "husband and wife" can be any two partners who are involved in cocreation, such as God and oneself, two lovers, unmarried partners, or close friends. The "children" can mean the creative results that spring from the cocreative acts of partnership.

I am He, you are She;
I am Song, you are Verse,
I am Heaven, you are Earth.
We two shall here together dwell,
becoming parents of children.

ATHARVA VEDA 14:2:71 (HINDUISM)

Sweet be the glances we exchange,
our faces showing true concord.
Enshrine me in your heart and let
one spirit dwell within us.

ATHARVA VEDA 7:36

The verse, "And Isaac brought her into his mother Sarah's tent" (Gen. 24:67), our masters have interpreted to mean that the Divine Presence came into Isaac's house along with Rebecca. According to the secret doctrine, the supernal Mother is together with the male only when the house is in readiness and at the time the male and female are conjoined. At such time blessings are showered forth by the supernal Mother upon them.

ZOHAR, GEN. 101B (JUDAISM)

Blessed art Thou, O Lord our God, King of the Universe, who has created all things to His Glory. . . .

May you be glad and exultant, O barren one, when her children are gathered to her with joy. Blessed art Thou, O Lord, who makes Zion joyful through her children.

May Thou make joyful these beloved companions, just as Thou gladdened Thy creatures in the Garden of Eden in primordial times. Blessed art Thou, O Lord, who make bridegroom and bride to rejoice.

Blessed art Thou, O Lord, King of the Universe, who created mirth and joy, bridegroom and bride, gladness, jubilation, dancing and delight, love and brotherhood, peace and fellowship. Quickly, O Lord our God, may the sound of mirth and joy be heard in the streets of Judah and Jerusalem, the voice of bridegroom and bride, jubilant voices of bridegrooms from their canopies and youths from the feasts of song. Blessed art Thou, O Lord, who makes the bridegroom rejoice with the bride.

TALMUD, KET. 8A (JUDAISM)

Among His signs is that He created spouses for you among yourselves that you may console yourselves with them. He has planted affection and mercy between you.

QURAN 30:21 (ISLAM)

A good wife who can find?
She is far more precious than jewels.
The heart of her husband trusts in her, and she will have
*   no lack of gain.*
She does him good, and not harm, all the days of her life. . . .
She opens her mouth with wisdom, and the teaching of
*   kindness is on her tongue. . . .*
Give her of the fruit of her hand, and let her works praise
*   her in the gates.*

PROV. 31:10–12, 26, 31

Greater love has no man than this: that a man lay down his life for his friends. You are my friends if you do what I command you. . . . This I command you, to love one another.

JOHN 15: 13–14, 17

Follow the scriptural readings of your choice with this prayer ritual:

Father-Mother Creator, ever-living Lord, it is right that we always and everywhere give you thanks. You, Lord, entered into a new covenant with your people. You restored us to grace through the healing mystery of Redemption. You gave us a share in the divine life through union with the energy of the Christ. You made us heirs of your eternal glory. This outpouring of love in the new covenant of grace is symbolized in the partnership covenant I now celebrate, which seals the love of Creator and His/Her creation and reflects your divine plan of loving mercy and kindness. And so with the angels and all the saints in heaven, we proclaim your glory and join in their unending hymn of praise. Thanks, praise, and glory be yours, now and forever. Amen.

You may conclude by performing the communion service or making the sign of the cross or blessing yourself with oil or water.

TEN

THE HOLY SPIRIT AS THE ENERGY MANIFESTATION OF GOD

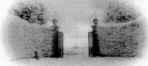

When I was forty-two years and seven months old, Heaven was opened and a fiery light of exceeding brilliance came and permeated my whole brain, and inflamed my whole heart and my whole breast, not like a burning but like a warming flame, as the sun warms anything its rays touch. And immediately I knew the meaning of the exposition of the Scriptures, namely the Psalter, the Gospel, and the other catholic volumes of both the Old and New Testaments, though I did not have the interpretation of the words of their texts or the division of the syllables or the knowledge of cases and tenses. But I had sensed in myself wonderfully the power and mystery of secret and admirable visions from my childhood—that is, from the age of five— up to that time, as I do now. This, however, I showed to no one except a few religious persons who were living in the same manner as I.

◆

HILDEGARD OF BINGEN, *SCIVIAS*

Anyone who has been raised in the Christian tradition or has even a passing acquaintance with it knows that the Holy Spirit is the Third Person of the Trinity. The name "Holy Spirit" replaced "Holy Ghost" during the 1950s and '60s because "Ghost" was considered to be spiritually incorrect. Christians aren't supposed to believe in ghosts, the spirits of the departed; and besides, the word has overtones of insubstantiality. But the name change did little to infuse more palpable meaning into the identity behind the words. Many Christians still wonder who or what exactly is the Holy Spirit.

One problem in identifying the Spirit is that the name has become synonymous to some extent with a stereotypical aspect of Pentecostalism. "When the Holy Spirit falls upon you," in born-again parlance, people jump up, clap their hands, start speaking in tongues, and engage in other emotional expressions. Those may or may not be manifestations of the Holy Spirit, but they are surely not the Holy Spirit. That's why Kathryn Kuhlman wouldn't allow speaking in tongues at her meetings, even though she was deeply Pentecostal. She felt that what many people claim to be the Holy Spirit is nothing more than a manifestation of their own emotion. "Some people think that noise is power," Kuhlman used to say, "and if that's true, then the Model-A Ford was the most powerful car ever built!"

Another problem in understanding what the Holy Spirit is derives from the classical terminology of the Trinity as "Three Persons in One God." Maybe it would have been better to call them three manifestations, because trying to think of the Holy Spirit as a person, as an individual of some sort, only confuses matters.

To begin with, this Spirit is called Holy because God is holy and God's desire for each of us is that we be whole. The root for the English word "holy" is the same as the root for "whole," and that root word also means "healthy." When the Holy Spirit, or the spirit of wholeness, is allowed to encompass every part of our being, especially from the inside out (which I call, aptly, holistic spirituality), then our spirit becomes deified—that is, more God-like—and from our spirit flows the Spirit of God to deify our soul, mind, emotions, and body. This has nothing to do with sin or the lack of sin in the traditional sense. It has everything to do with our openness and desire for the Spirit of the living God to dwell in us and work through us.

Each of us carries the presence of God within us wherever we go, but for most of us this Spirit lies dormant. For some, however, the power of the Spirit flows in a higher degree because they have become more conscious of it through prayer. In one whose prayer life has reached a state of perfect communion with the Father, as it did in Jesus, the presence is so powerful that merely by putting oneself in his proximity and remaining open to receiving God's grace, one can be healed. That's why the woman who came up and touched the hem of Jesus' garment experienced a presence powerful enough to heal her. The electromagnetic energy of the Spirit of God operating in Jesus passed directly through his clothes to the woman. That was the working of the Holy Spirit, and it's important to note that Jesus did not actually "heal" anyone, but only served as a conduit through whom the Father's healing energy was able to move unimpeded. Even the most gifted healers do not heal or perform "miracles"; the presence of God in them does the "miraculous" work. Once we know this, prayers take on a power that makes it possible to lift the world to a higher consciousness.

A year from now, if you remain committed to a life of prayer and communion with God, and stay open to the working of His Holy Spirit within you, your consciousness ought to expand beyond what it is today. You should also manifest a greater hunger and thirst as you become aware that life is more than what appears on the level of matter. Because we are made in the image of God, we are continually pulled toward an inner desire to develop a God-consciousness. Saint Paul says it well in his letter to the Ephesians: "I want to be filled full with the Spirit of Christ, the Spirit of God, with God himself." That's not symbolism, but the deep yearning of a person who is hungry for God.

In a footnote to the exchange between Yogananda and Therese Neumann which I quoted in the previous chapter, Yogananda adds his own gloss to Matthew 4:4 ("Man does not live by bread alone, but by every word that proceeds from the mouth of God"), insightfully tying together Eastern and Western conceptions of the power of the Holy Spirit. "Man's body battery," he writes,

> is not sustained by gross food (bread) alone, but by the vibratory cosmic energy (Word, or *Aum*). The invisible power flows into the human body through the gate of the medulla oblongata. This sixth bodily center is located at the back of the neck at the top of the five spinal *chakras* (Sanskrit for "wheels" or centers of radiating life force).

Yogananda goes on to draw further parallels between the Indian system of chakras, which I discussed briefly in Chapter 8, and the biblical understanding of the Holy Spirit:

> The medulla, the principal entrance for the body's supply of universal life energy (*Aum*), is directly connected

by polarity with the Christ Consciousness center [or third eye] in the single eye between the eyebrows: the seat of man's power of will. Cosmic energy is then stored up in the seventh center, in the brain, as a reservoir of infinite potentialities (mentioned in the *Vedas* as the "thousand-petaled lotus of light"). The Bible refers to *Aum* as the Holy Ghost or invisible life force that divinely upholds all creation. "What? know ye not that your body is the temple of the Holy Ghost which is in you, which ye have of God, and ye are not your own?" (1 Cor. 6:19).

In Eastern thought, Aum, or Om, is both a manifestation of spiritual power and a symbol of the presence of the Absolute within the material world. In that regard, Om is the Eastern counterpart of the Holy Spirit as the animating force of God's presence in the world.

Seen in these terms, the practice of prayer and fasting by certain mystics springs from a desire to know more of God by eliminating bread and focusing solely on the Word. John Lake, who was responsible for more than 100,000 healings in the Spokane, Washington, area in the early part of the twentieth century, describes it in this manner in his book about his life and faith:

> I went into fasting and prayer and waiting on God for nine months. And one day the glory of God in a new manifestation and a new incoming came to my life. When the phenomenon had passed and the glory of it remained in my soul, I found that my life began to manifest in the varied range of the gifts, given by the spirit, the very presence of God. . . . God flowed through

me with a new force. Healings were of a more powerful order. God lived in me; God manifested in me; God spoke through me. My spirit was deified.

Lake goes on to describe the results of prayer and fasting:

Then a new wonder manifested. My nature became so sensitized that I could lay hands on any man or woman and tell what organ was diseased, and to what extent, and all about it. I tested it. I went into hospitals where physicians could not diagnose a case, touched a patient, and instantly I knew the organ that was diseased, its extent, condition and location.

That is what it truly means to be filled with the Spirit.

Edgar Cayce, who worked somewhat differently, was able to go into a trance when he received a communication from someone who was sick, and in that trance he would give his diagnosis, naming the organ that was diseased and the way it could be healed. Sitting nearby, his wife or secretary would write down what he received from the spiritual dimension to send these people the results of the "reading."

We cannot limit how the Holy Spirit will work or through which people. In his book *Sister Aimee,* Daniel Epstein writes about the first major healing that took place with Aimee Semple McPherson. McPherson had already experienced what she called the "Baptism of the Holy Spirit," which she described as being like holding on to a large battery until the current became so powerful that every part of her body began to tremble. Subsequently, McPherson was approached by a young woman named Louise Messnick, who was suffering with advanced stages of rheumatoid arthritis. The inflammation had so impaired Messnick's neck muscles and jaw that she could not lift her head and could hardly chew.

> The vertebrae of her neck were skewed with the swelling and the ligaments of her back had begun to shorten so she could not stand erect. For a long time she had not been able to lift her hands high enough to comb her hair. Her fingers were gnarled and twisted.

Upon seeing the woman, Aimee cried out, "O Lord, you are able to heal her!" McPherson, the text continues,

> decided in that instant to pray for the crippled girl to be healed, but she would do it as inconspicuously as possible during the altar call. She would slip down to the front seat and pray quietly with her. In the back of her mind she thought that if Louise was not completely healed, the failure would be less noticeable. But the young cripple had whispered to her friend to carry her up at the very beginning of the altar call. Aimee gasped as she saw the young woman being carried to the front with all eyes upon her. Since she could not kneel, they sat her down in the central minister's chair high up for everyone to see.

Sister Aimee had called all these people together in the presence of the Holy Spirit for an anointing and an infusion of the divine presence. In her mind she carried a blueprint of the human body in radiant health. This is the way Aimee, Agnes Sanford, and many spiritual healers "see" the people they are working with. We do not focus on the sickness. We do not see them in the human form they're wearing at this particular time of their travels, but rather their authentic spiritual selves.

> She laid hands upon the woman's head. As she did this she felt an energy surge like an electric charge coming up from her heels right through her spine into her fingertips. The woman's cheeks flushed and her heartbeat increased. Aimee told her to lift up her hands and praise the Lord. Louise Messnick looked at her hands, lifted them up. And as she lifted them up some people in the front gasped with wonder. The hands unfolded from their claw-like deformity and straightened out. The hands went up until the arms were nearly straight above her head. She moved slowly along the rail hand over hand. And with every step she took, her limbs straightened. The fingers clutching the rail unknotted. Louise Messnick walked out of the church that night alone, without her crutches.

Despite the clear connection between prayer and healing through the power of the Holy Spirit, in our desire to know God and experience that power we often do everything *except* pray. We genuinely want to experience the essence of God, which the scriptures call signs and wonders, or spiritual phenomena, but we are not sure how to go about it. Prayer is the quickest and most reliable vehicle to help open our hearts to the action of the Holy Spirit. But what precisely is the nature of that Spirit?

In early mystical writings, the universe was seen as a womb to be impregnated by the Breath of God to become alive. Mystical religions invest a lot of time in trying to understand the concept of breath in its fullest dimension, especially its spiritual dimension, because mystics see Spirit as the Breath of God. God continually breathes His own life force, via the Spirit, into everything. In Genesis, the creative Breath of God generates life. Later the Breath would be described as "Holy Spirit," "Spirit of God," or "Spirit of the Christ." Saint Paul spoke about this all-powerful Breath of God when he said that the same divine energy that raised Jesus from the dead is in each of us to "quicken" our mortal bodies, that is, to make our bodies well and to make us congruent with our spirit and our soul.

The Holy Spirit, then, is the divine primordial energy released in the universe through God's will. When Jesus was talking to the Samaritan woman, she began a discussion on the worship of God, to which Jesus responded, "God is Spirit." It follows that if you want to worship God, you must worship God from a spiritual dimension, from the inside of your being with love in any place at any time, for God is everywhere. By saying this, Jesus affirmed the fact that God cannot be localized. Yet religion has repeatedly attempted to localize God. "This is where you'll find Him," those of a certain sect will say; "my way is the only true path." Yet Jesus makes it very clear: God is Spirit, and like the wind, the spirit blows wherever it will. Like fire, the spirit will consume whatever the spirit desires.

In his book *Desert Wisdom*, Neil Douglas-Klotz quotes and expands on several passages from the Aramaic Peshitta, the ancient Aramaic text of the Gospels to which I've already referred. The following is from John 3:3–8:

> Niqadimaw [Nicodemus], a Pharisee, came to Isho'a [Jesus] at night and said to him Teacher, we know that you are sent from Alaha, the Source, because no one can do what you are doing unless the Source is with him. Isho'a answered and said, "By the earth on which we stand, what I am going to say is the ground of truth and

the source from which my actions grow. [In other words, what I am about to say to you is the truth upon which I stand and live.] Unless one is born again, that one cannot enter the kingdom of God. Unless a human being is completely regenerated [think of "regenerated" not in theological terms but scientifically], propagated, and reborn of the Center of existence, from the primal origin of light and fire [Holy Spirit], that person will not see the sudden vision, be illuminated by the flash, the 'I Can' of the Cosmos, the creative fire of the soul's source."

When you read these words you may be confused about their meaning. For example, to be "illuminated by the flash" refers to the intuitive awareness that comes to you when you are connected with the Spirit of God, the "I can" of the Cosmos. Jesus is saying that people have lost the awareness that they are made in the image of the eternal "I can." If they are aware that they are made in the image of God and carry the primordial energy of the Spirit, nothing is impossible for that God-presence within them.

Every time you change the word "can" to "can't," you are taking the name of the Lord in vain. God is saying "I can," and because God created you and me out of the essence of ability, then that is to be our vocabulary also. Apply that principle to your prayer. Are your prayers based on "I can"—or "I think I can" or "I can't"? God never said, "I think there ought to be light."

In the Aramaic Peshitta version of John's Gospel, Nicodemus pressures Jesus further, inquiring as to how one can be born when one is old. Can one enter the second time into his mother's womb and be born? Jesus assures Nicodemus that it is possible to be born again by returning to the essence of one's eternal nature, which is spirit, and entering into a relationship with the Source of all life, the Breath of life, Holy Spirit.

In speaking to the Roman Christians, Saint Paul told them to live their life according to the Spirit, not according to the flesh. Unfortunately, the Christian Church's fear of sexuality plays into a reading of this translation that makes it seem as if what we have to guard against are the desires of the flesh. I think we can better understand this truth if we interpret the word "flesh" as "ego," if by ego we understand that separative aspect of the self that seeks personal survival above all else. Seen in these terms, the real battle of life is not between sexuality and celibacy but between spirit and ego.

I would therefore paraphrase Romans 8:5–6 to read like this: "For those who live according to the ego set their minds on the things of the ego, but those who live according to the Spirit set their minds on the things of the Spirit. To set the mind on ego is death, but to set the mind on the Spirit is life and peace."

The ego, or survival instinct, diminishes us as spiritual beings. Spirit, on the other hand, keeps us in tune with our authentic essence: the creative result of the Breath of God. To expand our prayer life and draw maximum energy from all our prayers, we need to heighten our awareness of the Holy Spirit as God's inspiration continually at work within us. This represents a subtle but significant extension of our previous work to maintain an awareness of and connection with God throughout the day.

INVOCATION OF THE HOLY SPIRIT

The Holy Spirit, by definition in Genesis, is the emanating power of Breath, the expression of the Source. God has traditionally revealed Himself to the mystics as the Source of all life. At certain times of the day, then, it is beneficial for us to be aware of our breathing and remind ourselves that "God is." When we eat or drink, it is also beneficial to our spiritual growth to remind ourselves, "God is the Source of this food and drink." As we are walking outdoors, it can be of great benefit to remind ourselves, "God is the Source of all life, including these trees, these flowers, this rain, this snow, those birds, that sunset." Once you consciously become aware of the movement of God's Holy Spirit in and around you, your prayer life will be enhanced remarkably.

At other times, you may say the following prayer, focusing your attention and praying slowly from the heart. Feel free to substitute this prayer for others that you may have begun repeating throughout the course of the day. While saying it, however, whether silently or aloud, pay special attention to the intake and outflow of your breath, being aware that the breath itself carries the Spirit of God within you:

Come, Holy Spirit, bring me your wisdom and understanding.

Come, Holy Spirit, help me experience the Father's love.

Come, Holy Spirit, help me see Jesus more clearly, walk with him more closely, love him more dearly.

Come, Holy Spirit, help me see your essence in the many images of the sacred on earth, including Kuan Yin, Shiva, the Buddha, and Mother Mary. Help me find you in the face of Tara, Lao-tzu, Confucius, and Xangô. Show me your workings in the person of Ramana Maharshi, Mother Meera, Buffalo Calf Woman, and other manifestations of your Divine Presence.

Come, Holy Spirit, shower your gifts upon me, manifest especially your gift of healing.

Come, Holy Spirit, reveal to me my need for God, my need to seek first His kingdom, His way of holiness, then I know all else shall be added.

Come, Holy Spirit, spirit of prayer, help me praise and worship my Lord who loves me so much.

Come, Holy Spirit, break down the barriers within me that keep me from experiencing the God who is all good.

Come, Holy Spirit, teach me love, teach me true joy, teach me peace that I may always be your vessel of life to others.

Come, Holy Spirit, come!

By increasing our awareness of the Holy Spirit's presence at work in the world, we also become more attuned to the consequences of that work. We can begin by gleaning intimations of those consequences from the two most prominent passages in the Judeo-Christian scriptures regarding the Holy Spirit, both of which are found near the end of the Old Testament. In Zechariah 4:6, God speaks to Zerubbabel, the leader of His people, reminding Zerubbabel that it will not be by human power that he will conquer: "Not by might, nor by power, but by my spirit, saith the Lord of hosts." What God was saying to Zerubbabel he is also saying to us: Not by your own might or your own strength, not even by your own mind or wisdom will you bring an end to any strife or problems you are experiencing. The only way that struggle will end is through experiencing the presence of God's Spirit in your life. To the followers of God, the message is clear: No more are you to live in your own power but in God's.

In the second Chapter of the Book of Joel, which would later be quoted by Peter in his opening sermon after Pentecost (Acts 2:16ff), God promises that His own life and energy will be permanently available to all the people. "And it shall come to pass afterward, that I will pour out my spirit upon all flesh; and your sons and your daughters shall prophesy, your old men shall dream dreams, your young men shall see visions. And also upon the servants and upon the handmaids in those days will I pour out my spirit" (2:28–29). This is essentially a restatement and rephrasing of God's wish to Moses in Exodus that His people should be "a kingdom of priests and a holy nation." But what is especially significant is the inclusive language: "your sons *and your daughters* shall prophesy. . . ." Despite the best efforts of the Jewish and Christian hierarchies to limit women or completely exclude them from prominent roles in spiritual life, scripture does not back them up.

Just as the Israelites lost sight of God's desire in the pre-Christian era, so the Christian Church has also lost sight of His wishes as expressed in the very scripture both Jews and Christians revere. But as with the Jewish people, Christianity has had its share of mystics and visionaries in whose inner eye God's desire has burned brightly at times. In the twelfth century, to cite one example, lived a marvelous mystic by the name of Hildegard of Bingen, who was not only a prophetess but also a healer and a visionary who had a powerful experience of the dynamic Spirit of God. When people came to her with their illnesses, she would offer prayer, making available to them the presence and power of the Holy Spirit. Hildegard would ask the Holy Spirit what medicine these people could take for their healing. And in much the same way as it was to happen for Edgar Cayce many centuries later, the Spirit spoke to her in visions and dreams and told her what herbs and combinations of herbs she could use or recommend to these people for the continued maintenance of their healing.

In his book *Illuminations of Hildegard of Bingen,* Matthew Fox writes that "Hildegard does not hesitate to appropriate the Pentecost experience, the Spirit's fire that illumines and thaws and connects, to herself. It was when she was 'inflamed by a fiery light' that she put her hand to writing. . . . [D]octrine for Hildegard is not primarily an object to be studied but the naming of an experience undergone."

The reverse of Hildegard's experience appears to be true today. In wanting to have our theology correct, we have become so submerged in doctrine and dogma that we miss the presence and Spirit of God. For Hildegard, doctrine was only an attempt at explaining one's experience, one's personal identification with the Spirit of God, whether that experience be prophecy, visions, or miraculous healings.

"And like the first recipients of this spirit in the Book of Acts," Fox continues,

> the power of the spirit's awakening is not meant for oneself but for others. The first disciples, like Hildegard, were cured of their doubt and fear so as to preach Good News to Parthians, Medes and Elamites. . . . And so Hildegard too begins her missionary activity, her being sent to the church to speak of its own inner beauty and also its corruption.
>
> In picturing herself as the recipient of the Pentecostal fire, Hildegard is also and once again talking of her prophetic vocation. Peter got up on that first Pentecost day and declared that the disciples were not drunk as was plainly thought (Hildegard has been called crazy many times over the centuries). Rather the disciples— read Hildegard—were fulfilling the words of the prophet Joel.

In effect, Hildegard was saying to those in the hierarchy in her day, "I, along with all women, am just as important as the Apostles and disciples were at Pentecost." As Fox points out, Hildegard "is counting herself among these recipients of the dynamic spirit of God." So must we.

God empowers us with love, with peace, with joy, and with

strength. But this empowerment is all internal, and that's where we so often make our error. Internal power works from the inside out, but it is not a power that you can grasp from the outside and bring in to you. This power is released through our connection with God and what I have been calling prayer and the various aspects of prayer, especially meditation or contemplation.

From the earliest times, God planned for his people to be spirit-governed, meaning that they would live their lives through the guidance of the Holy Spirit. God would shepherd his people and be their provision and their peace. They would need fear nothing so long as they realized that they were made in God's image—Spirit. God's children soon began to move in another direction, however, away from the Spirit and toward the material. People no longer believed and trusted in prophecy, visions, or miracles. Their manifestations of the Spirit began to disappear from view. Fortunately, people today are recognizing that there is more to life than struggling and even dying for material wealth. Many are returning to the awareness that we are all spirit and so are interconnected with each other and our Source.

In a way quite differently from how many fundamentalist Christians believe it, I believe this era is experiencing the Second Coming of Christ. The spirit of the Christ begins to fill the whole world as the days of "country club" religion slowly come to a close and a new era dawns in our awareness—that of the Holy Spirit dwelling among all the people of God. Today it seems that what we refer to as "spiritual phenomena" are occurring all over the world. Some people have difficulty believing these manifestations; yet I find it hard to understand why so many people who call themselves religious can't accept these phenomena, labeling them as the work of the devil or demons.

When we look at mystical phenomena, we ought to look beyond the manifestations of God and see only God. We must learn to say to ourselves, "I want to develop a relationship with God. I want to experience God." Often some unusual phenomenon will be the catalyst to draw us more deeply into God-awareness. But we must be careful never to emphasize spiritual phenomena apart from God, as if you could have a "mystical experience" without God. The experience itself is simply a manifestation of God's Spirit at work. This lesson was powerfully driven home to me some ten years ago when I began to visit the site of many startling spiritual phenomena: the town of Medjugorje in Eastern Europe.

By 1985, I had already been involved with spiritual healing work for ten years, yet I was quite aware that something was missing from my life. Although I had witnessed many people being healed or cured instantly from various maladies as a result of my ministrations, my own life seemed to be disintegrating more and more. Around this time, my associate in the healing work, Paul Funfsinn, returned from a stay in the tiny village of Medjugorje in the country of Bosnia, part of the former Yugoslavia. Paul shared with me his startling experience of supernatural phenomena taking place there in the form of apparitions of the Blessed Virgin Mary. At that time, I was still a Roman Catholic priest pastoring a small country parish, and like most Midwesterners, Catholic or not, I found it hard to believe in apparitions. Paul planned to return to Medjugorje, and after much persuasion, I decided to go along. I did not intend to be caught up in a "spiritual high," but I did believe that being in such a place might help me to discover and fulfill God's will for me.

We arrived in Medjugorje on a weekday and I could immediately sense the extraordinary spiritual character of the place. On the surface, it was just a typical Eastern European village, poor and picturesque. Yet friendliness and love permeated its atmosphere. As I was roaming the streets near the Church of St. James shortly after arriving, a Catholic nun who worked with the visionaries—the youngsters who were said to be seeing Mary—approached and asked me if I would like to be part of the small gathering of folks joining the visionaries at the time of Mary's next apparition.

"Indeed, yes!" I shouted, delighted and a bit surprised at this kind and completely unsolicited offer. Entering the room with the others, I found a spot where I could be comfortable. The "apparition room" was nothing more than a tiny cell in the home of the Franciscan priests who were serving the parish. While we waited, some knelt and prayed the rosary. I prayed, but remained seated in my chair. The visionaries entered the room along with one of the priests and the nun who had invited me, and stood together at one end of the cell. For some reason, I began to move slowly off my chair and onto my knees. After a few moments, the three of them then dropped to the floor on their knees. Just as they did, a bright light appeared like a bolt of lightning. Although Paul had given me some general sense of what was going on in Medjugorje, he hadn't told me that it always began with a blinding flash of light. I was completely unprepared, and when the light came it knocked me off my knees and threw me against the wall! I found myself lying on the ground, my head under a low table.

Convinced that I had made a fool of myself and that people must be staring at me, I lay there immobile for several minutes, afraid to open my eyes. When I mustered the courage to look around, I discovered that no one was paying the least attention to me. They had probably seen it all before. And besides, they were too busy praying to regard a poor egotist. At the end of the session, I left the room bewildered, not knowing that what had just occurred was about to transform me and my work forever. That was one hell of a wake-up call!

The next few days passed in a fog, although my experiences

were deeply moving. The chain of a new crystal rosary I had purchased prior to my departure had turned gold—apparently a "normal" phenomenon among many of the visitors to Medjugorje, I was later informed. I saw plenty of phenomena, even though I had not been looking for them. In the room where priests celebrated mass for the people coming to the village was a large statue of Mary, and Paul and I observed an image of the Christ suddenly appear in light on the statue's breast. Paul captured it in a photograph, although the image disappeared from the statue. Along with the others, we were able to stare at the sun without hurting our eyes as it danced and pulsated, overlaid with what appeared to be a large whole-wheat wafer like a communion host. On the left of this image was the kneeling figure of the Blessed Virgin.

I tried to take these things calmly, telling myself again that I was here only to discover God's will for me and not to be "wowed" by spiritual phenomena, although, at the very least, I had been given quite a lot to digest. I returned home inflamed with a new outlook on my life and my work. The change, I can see now, was the result of something that had occurred on an inner level. It may have been related to the phenomena in the sense of having happened simultaneously with them, but it did not come as a result of witnessing them. All I knew was that something important was happening there, for me just as for many other souls, and I had to return to find out more about it.

My second visit to Medjugorje took place only six months later. Between 1985 and 1988, I was guided to make four trips in all to this remarkable sacred site—apparently I'm a slow learner. During the course of the other three trips, astonishing things continued to happen. The chain of a blue crystal rosary, which I had owned for a long time, also turned gold. I witnessed more light phenomena and, after returning home again, some extraordinary manifestations of the sun spinning over my own parish in Illinois.

This happened one evening prior to a healing service and was witnessed by over fifty attendees.

Still, during all my pilgrimages, I wasn't really focused on the external phenomena. I kept returning to my original question: What was God's will for me?

After meditating for some time on the events that surrounded my journeys to this isolated European village, a number of deeply disturbing revelations were given to me that would enhance the course of my life from this time forward. I was informed by a voice within my spirit, for instance, that I had been too "hard" in dealing with people who were sick and in need of help. Although God's Spirit was able to heal them through me, my lack of compassion was closing the channel for me to experience the same joy that people were feeling through their communion with God. I was also told that I lacked the qualities of the feminine energy of God— namely, tenderness and mercy—that Mary, the Mother of Jesus, symbolized. I had become so busy with the work of the Lord that I had forgotten the Lord of the work.

As I meditated further on Jesus, Mary, the Holy Spirit, and the Christ-consciousness, the realization came that God could mold me into the image of love, mercy, tenderness, strength, and power that described the compassionate human being. Recognizing God as a God of love is the beginning of a profound wisdom that enables one to rise above the seeming tragedies of life into the very heart of God as both Mother and Father, which is the God Jesus knew. Mary and Jesus demonstrate the completeness of feminine and masculine energy in the "personality" of God. Somehow the Holy Spirit was working in me to achieve this (for me) new vision of the Divine.

These events and revelations empowered my personal life and healing work in a deeply moving way. I am now able, through the Holy Spirit, to be a clearer channel for God's presence and power in my own life as well as to give others a God not only of power but of tenderness, care, and mercy. I believe it is dangerous for people without spiritual awareness and a desire for authentic spiritual growth to try to develop psychic powers. Just about anyone who sets his mind to it and works diligently can develop such powers, but if you don't also pursue spiritual growth, you're asking for trouble. This is not because God is going to "get" you, but because you are attempting to set yourself into a dimension of living that will damage you on a psychic or physical level or both. Indian mystics have long warned their followers of the danger of what they call *siddhis,* psychic powers ranging from levitation to bilocation. Although these may be byproducts of a diligent dedication to meditative practices, they can be, at best, a distraction from the spiritual path. At worst, they can lead one into all kinds of ego-deluded blind alleys.

Spiritual phenomena are manifestations of the Holy Spirit and are not for the purpose of entertainment; they are to be accepted humbly for the good of all. The high-voltage energy contained in healing work is to be used for that purpose only. To use it unwisely will cause the energy to "backfire," eventually consuming the vessel through whom it comes. Tapping the energy of the Holy Spirit, Jesus healed, multiplied loaves and fishes, produced a coin out of a fish's mouth, practiced clairvoyance and clairaudience, was illuminated (during the Transfiguration), and levitated (at the Ascension). The beauty of these events lies not in the phenomena themselves but in the fact that Jesus said we could do these things too—and more—through the reception of the Spirit into our lives.

The Holy Spirit is the key to understanding the significance of all spiritual phenomena. When the people asked Saint Peter to tell them about his Master, he said, "Jesus was anointed by God with the Holy Spirit." Jesus began his work by declaring, "The Spirit of the Lord God is upon me." Jesus of Nazareth told his followers that they were to do what he himself did and that Jesus would assist them by releasing the Holy Spirit, the divine energy of God, at a specific time. That this release would be ushered in by physical manifestations would serve to make them conscious of their empowerment, an empowerment that would enable them to love one another genuinely, as Jesus loved—no hidden agenda allowed! Their empowerment had nothing to do with their worthiness or lack of it. It was a matter of grace. God would grace them so that they could see themselves as God sees them, as sons and daughters, recognizing that not only were they one with God, but also that all God had was available for them.

God's plan for our fullness in life is still in effect. Our work will consist of learning how to tune in to God through prayer, thereby receiving the Spirit and then releasing that same Spirit into a world hungry to experience firsthand the energy of God's love.

PRAYER TO THE HOLY SPIRIT

I have said that silent prayer—opening the heart to catch the thoughts of God—is the highest form of authentic prayer. Yet we often find it helpful to use language to prepare ourselves for entry into this state. I hope that you will find the words I've provided useful, but I also want to encourage you to create prayers of your own. By way of example, here is a prayer that I created some time ago, based on the prayer to the Holy Spirit quoted earlier in this chapter. I had fashioned that prayer, in turn, from a few phrases that appeared in an old prayer book. By watching how I have expanded and improvised on the basic language of invoking the Holy Spirit, perhaps you can create a prayer of your own around the same premise. Then return to other prayers in this book (or in the Appendixes at the end) and work with them in a similar fashion.

Come, Holy Spirit: Replace my restless, tense mind with the peace that comes from knowing there is a Guide who leads me into the tranquil valley, where He refreshes me with fertile, lovely, inspiring, uplifting thoughts.

Replace the anxiety and fear within me, O Lord, with the calm serenity, quiet confidence, and courageous faith that comes from knowing there is a Rock upon whom I am able to lean during the storm—a Rock that will not falter or crumble, a Rock that is sturdy and strong, the Spirit of the Christ who is always there, waiting with arms outstretched.

Replace the scars of bitterness and resentment within me with the ointment of joy and gladness that comes from knowing the Forgiver and Healer who wraps me in His tender care ever so lovingly, as a gentle father embraces his newborn child.

Replace the coldness and hardness of my heart, the dullness of my mind, the darkness of my spirit, with the soft, warm, golden rays of your never-ending Light. Penetrate down deep into my very being, uncovering all that was hidden, and enliven within me once again the dying ember of a great love for God, for others, and myself.

Lord God, thank you for letting me see myself as you see me, a wonderful being made in your image, vibrant and alive with abilities and potential for doing great things for you and your people.

Lord, thank you for this tremendous, powerful truth that you are with me and for me all the days of my life, healing me and filling me full of your Holy Spirit, a Spirit of Love, Peace, and Joy.

ELEVEN

PRAYER AS BLESSING AND DECREE

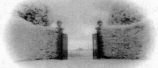

Thou shalt also decree a thing, and it shall be established unto thee: and the light shall shine upon thy ways.

◆

JOB 22:28

Perhaps the most telling episode in the Gospels connecting prayer with the power to heal comes in Chapter 9 of the Gospel of Mark, which relates the events surrounding the Transfiguration of Jesus. According to that passage (this and the excerpts that follow are from *The Amplified Bible*, 1965),

> Jesus took with him Peter and John and James, and went up on a high mountain, apart by themselves. And he was transfigured before them and became resplendent with divine brightness. And his garments became glistening, intensely white, as no fuller (cloth dresser) on earth could bleach them. And Elijah appeared there to them, accompanied by Moses, and they were holding (a protracted) conversation with Jesus.

At this point Peter, who "did not really know what to say, for they were in a violent fright—aghast [with] dread" suggests setting up a kind of memorial on the spot: three tents, one each for Jesus, Moses, and Elijah. No wonder Peter ended up being the first head of the church hierarchy: something amazing and ineffable occurs and he wants to build a monument to it! But at that moment a cloud overshadows them and a voice is heard echoing the voice that spoke after Jesus was baptized by John in the River Jordan, saying, "This is my beloved Son; listen to him."

After this extraordinary event, the four of them descend from the mountain and join up with the disciples.

> And when they came to the nine disciples, they saw a great crowd around them, and scribes questioning and

disputing with them. And immediately all of the crowd when they saw Jesus (returning from the holy mountain, his face and person yet glistening) were greatly amazed and ran up to him and greeted him. And he asked them, about what are you questioning and discussing with them? And one of the throng replied to him, Teacher, I brought my son to you, for he has a dumb spirit. And wherever it lays hold of him (so as to make him its own), it dashes him down and convulses him, and he foams (at the mouth) and grinds his teeth, and he (falls into a motionless stupor) and is wasting away; and I asked your disciples to drive it out, and they were not able.

At this point Jesus expresses his exasperation that his disciples haven't yet gleaned the kernel of truth in what he has been trying to teach them. "O unbelieving generation—without any faith!" he exclaims. "How long shall I (have to do) with you? How long am I to bear with you? Bring him to me."

The disciples still lack the kind of faith—the faith that Jesus has already told them is sufficient to move mountains—needed to heal the epileptic boy. When they bring the boy to Jesus, he asks the boy's father, "How long has he had this?"

The father answers, "From the time he was a little boy. And it has often thrown him both into fire and into water, intending to kill him; but if you can do anything, do have pity on us and help us."

Jesus is taken aback once again. "If you can do anything?" he asks incredulously. It's one of the great ironic moments in the Gospels. Clearly this man hasn't heard the full story, so Jesus reiterates his simple credo: "All things are possible to him who believes!"

"At once the father of the boy gave (an eager, piercing, inarticulate) cry with tears, and he said, Lord, I believe! Constantly help my weakness of faith!"

Jesus then proceeds to rebuke the spirit or spirits that possess the boy, who momentarily swoons and appears dead until Jesus takes him by the hand and lifts him up.

"And when he had gone indoors," the Gospel account continues, "his disciples asked him privately, Why could not we drive it out? And he replied to them, This kind cannot be driven out by anything but prayer" (Mark 9:2–4, 14–29).

Here it seems that Jesus is talking about a kind of prayer somewhat different from that which I've been describing throughout this book. We don't actually know how Jesus prayed when he was alone, since that was not recorded. We can, however, see the results. When Jesus went up the mountain to commune with God, he achieved such an intense union that he was quite literally illuminated—"flashing with the brilliance of lightning," according to one translation. His spiritual battery fully charged with light-energy from communion with the Father, Jesus descended and immediately performed a healing that was beyond the capability of his disciples.

When Jesus said, "This kind cannot be driven out by anything but prayer," I believe he was referring to more than just the transfigurative prayer through which he had become spiritually recharged. He may also have been talking specifically about a kind of prayer known as *decree*. From the many Gospel accounts of his healings, we can see that he practiced this form of prayer regularly. In its simplest form, decree is a command for something to come to be. In this case, Jesus rebuked the unclean spirit and commanded that it come out of the boy, as he had done earlier in the episode of the Gadarene demoniac (Mark 5:1–20). In other instances, he decreed that people who asked him for healing be healed, and they were. The level of faith and confidence required for such a decree to bear immediate fruit is obviously quite high—even the disciples Jesus had personally instructed hadn't yet reached this level. Although decreeing that a seriously ill person heal instantly may seem beyond the capabilities of most of us, an awareness of the syntax of decree will help our thinking with regard to prayer in general. In the meantime, as our faith grows, we can certainly practice a form of decree known as *blessing*.

For reasons that should be clear from my discussion of the Lord's Prayer, I'm not especially fond of prescribed prayer forms like the Hail Mary, the Apostles' Creed, or the Rosary. Yet some forms of prayer can be beneficial if they haven't been rendered virtually meaningless by years of rote repetition. Blessing is one such form, in which we call down God's divine favor upon people and circumstances, potentially releasing God's creative energy in a dynamic way.

A blessing is not a petition; it is not even an affirmation. A blessing is an actual event. Just by sitting down, relaxing, and pronouncing the word "peace," you can experience at least a subtly peaceful feeling, even if only for a split second. That's indicative of the energy of blessing, which to my mind is quite distinct from what is commonly referred to as affirmation. The difference is that affirmation literally means to attempt to make firm something that may not as yet be physically manifested. To affirm, for example, "I am now at my ideal weight and I have no difficulty staying there," when you are in fact fifty pounds overweight, is a form of wishful thinking. If you want to lose weight, you would do better to repeat, "I am a child of God." That way you would at least build up your self-esteem and self-awareness instead of trying to convince yourself that you have already lost the weight. Some forms of affirmation are fine because they simply state and reinforce the truth: "God loves me and wants me to prosper." I simply believe that blessing provides a much more potent way of doing the same thing.

Even if you feel that you'll never use blessing for healing

another person, either because that's not your calling or you're not comfortable with it, you can still learn how to use blessings for yourself. To begin, you can turn any statement into a blessing by calling it upon yourself in a simple way that is easy to master.

CREATING A BLESSING FROM SCRIPTURE

I'm convinced that if I show you how I create the kinds of prayers and blessings I've been sharing with you in this book, you will eventually learn how to create prayers and blessings on your own. Let me begin with a couple of examples drawn from working with the Psalms. Although not all the Psalms are equally appealing—many of them reflect the anguished cries of an oppressed people calling on God to smite their enemies—I often find them to be an excellent source of raw material from which to create blessings. You might just as easily, however, follow this procedure with writings from your favorite Buddhist, Hindu, or Taoist sacred texts, or from some of the excellent collections of religious myths from the African and Native American traditions.

For this example, I will begin by reading Psalm 34 (Psalm 33 in Catholic Bibles):

> I will bless the Lord at all times; his praise is always on my lips.
> In the Lord my soul shall make its boast; the humble shall hear
>   and be glad.
> Therefore glorify the Lord with me; together let us praise his
>   name!
> I sought the Lord and he answered me, from all my terrors he set
>   me free.
> Look toward him and be radiant; so your faces shall never be
>   ashamed.

oint in my reading, the word "radiant" captures my atten-
ke my prayer beads and with each bead, so that my body
will be coordinated with the thought coming in, I repeat the word
"radiant" until I begin to feel radiant myself. I could also go back to
the phrase "Therefore glorify the Lord with me" and turn it around
to say, "I glorify the Lord."

As you repeat the phrase you select, it can become a blessing. You may even feel a rushing in of warmth, although this may
be delicate at first if you are not aware of it. As you become alert to
the possibilities, sensations such as warmth or tingling may begin
to get stronger.

To take another example, let's use Psalm 62 (or 61), which
begins:

> In God alone is my soul at rest; my help comes from Him.
> God alone is my rock, my stronghold, my fortress; I stand firm.

To say "In God alone is my soul at rest" is itself a blessing. You are
not asking for help but are recognizing a state of being. Now let's
move to a line from the last verses of the Psalm (11b–12a): "To God
alone belongs power, and to you, Lord, love." You can take that
line, insert your own name, and change the wording slightly. I
would read it like this: "Ron, I bless you now with the power and
the love of God." By calling it down upon yourself, you are turning
a statement or an affirmation into a blessing.

If a woman is praying this Psalm, she should have no qualms
about substituting female pronouns for male. Say, "In God alone is
my soul at rest, my help comes from Her." At first this may feel
strange, but in the end it may well forge a greater divine connection on the blessing level.

I frequently follow the same procedure with scriptural passages. If God is talking to Moses and the Lord says something like,

"Tell the people I want to prosper them," I'll personalize it: "Ron, I want to prosper you." Now I've turned it into a blessing I can use anytime. If you have a favorite line or prayer from any tradition, begin with that. See if you can make a blessing out of it so that it is no longer just a helpful phrase to recall in times of crisis, but also an empowering incantation that can actively help you through a difficult moment. Take, for example, the classic line from the Buddhist Dhammapada (5): "Hatred is never appeased by hatred in this world; it is appeased by love. This is an eternal Law." At a moment when you feel strongly tempted to return hatred or anger for the hatred or anger of another, simply say, "I never appease hatred by hatred; I appease it by love."

Most of the prayers in the Old Testament are actually prayers of blessing, which was a favored form of prayer for the Jewish people and was often accompanied by specific rituals. Excluding instances where the root word for "bless" is used to mean "fortunate" or "happy," as in the Beatitudes, the words "blessing" or "blessed" occur over four hundred times in the Bible. Throughout the Old Testament, prophets, kings, and priests anointed and blessed the people while God manifested Himself in some form of energy such as light or fire. Since that time, to be sure, many religions have allowed blessing to degenerate into an empty ritual stripped of its inherent power. We can recapture the energy emitted from blessing, however, if we recall the essence and meaning of the act itself.

In keeping with our insights into the nature of authentic prayer, to bless does not mean to ask God to do something but instead to declare His intention and willingness to do it. In Chapter 6 of the Book of Numbers, for example, the priests received specific instructions from God as to how they were to bless the people of Israel, that is, to grace them with the energy of God. The Lord told Moses to instruct his progeny precisely how to phrase this blessing (6:24–26):

> *The Lord bless you, the Lord keep you:*
> *The Lord make his face to shine upon you, and the Lord*
> *   be gracious unto you:*
> *The Lord turn his face toward you and grant you peace.*

To put this in my own words, as I do when delivering the blessing myself, I would phrase it this way:

> *The Lord bless you and protect you.*
> *The Lord's face brighten with joy because of you.*
> *The Lord be gracious to you and favor you, granting you*
> *   peace.*

The Hebrew word *shalom,* translated here as "peace," involves more than just the absence of war. *Shalom* implies "wholeness" and "completeness": may everything and everyone you need to make your life abundantly full be yours.

By affirming either version of these words a few times either silently or aloud, you can begin to experience an energy coming forth from the words themselves and charging the atmosphere with the divine electricity of God. A vibration suffuses the prayer of blessing as it does prayers of decree, and it can carry a sacred energy and power out into the world to create good. This is an energy one does not experience in the prayer of petition, and for that reason alone it deserves a special place in your repertoire of sacred utterances.

Blessings are powerful conduits of spiritual energy. The main vehicle for the release of this creative energy is our speaking of words given to humanity by God. When you proclaim a blessing over a person or situation, you desire to bring forth the goodness inherent in that person or situation. By the act of blessing, you declare the good in a person or situation to be manifested. By so doing, the blesser is releasing the energy of God that already exists in the spiritual atmosphere to bring forth this good even in a condition that is perceived to be bad. When the ancient Hebrews spoke a blessing over their children and households, the benefits were immeasurable.

Blessings produce tangible experiences of energy vibrations. People on the giving and receiving end of blessings often feel a tingling sensation passing through their bodies as God's creative energy moves through them. In many forms of prayer, especially the prayers one was taught to memorize and say out of habit, one usually feels nothing at all. These prayers generally make very little connection with God, as the person praying most likely feels separated from God and so must cry out to a Being far off in another galaxy instead of discovering the God whose kingdom is within. Sadly, one praying in this fashion is not aware that he or she is a temple of divine energy, a temple of the Holy Spirit, or that the presence of the divine energy that raised Jesus from the dead is lying dormant within, awaiting resurrection.

That divine energy that lies within us, similar to what Indian adepts call the Kundalini energy that lies dormant at the base of the spine, I prefer to call "resurrection current." This current is spiritual electricity that causes people who have a loving connection with God to do what Jesus told his disciples to do, that is, to have their life, being, and movement in the Holy Spirit. The early followers of Jesus reached out to people, allowing the energy of God in that resurrection current to use them as channels for healing the sick and producing miracles, electrifying the very atmosphere around them. This is what happened to the woman with the hemorrhage who was healed by touching the hem of Jesus' garment. It occurred again when Jesus was transfigured and, aglow with the energy of God, his garment became breathtakingly white. We too can arrive at being aglow with the Spirit of God when our human spirit encounters the Divine. Blessing is one way to make this communion happen.

When I was involved in that automobile accident on the Los Angeles freeway described earlier, I was forced to learn the lesson regarding blessing as a positive energy force. At the time of the accident, blessing in the form of forgiveness was the furthest thought from my mind. In the following weeks, in fact, my anger turned into rage and my life began falling apart. The California Highway Patrol was unable to find the accident report, thereby rendering my car nonexistent and dashing any hope of a quick settlement and money to purchase a new car. Payment due me from hospital and car insurance was simply not forthcoming. I was overwhelmed with self-pity until a friend of mine suggested a practical approach to forgiveness in the form of blessing all concerned with thoughts of loving release. This sounded like a good idea until I tried to do it! Summoning my best powers of visualization to review the incident and pronounce the words "I forgive you and bless you with love," I still felt nothing but anger.

At this point, a pastor I knew from the Assembly of God suggested that I set up what he called a blessing table. This can be any small table or shelf, or just a pillow on the floor in front of you, on which you place the things that are frustrating you at the moment. Since I'm an analytical person who needs to concretize my feelings, I immediately responded to his suggestion. I put all the paperwork, letters from my insurance company, and photos of the wrecked car on a little folding table in the room where I prayed. At first I actually became more annoyed by looking at my ruined car. Then I placed a small votive candle in front of the pictures, and put a crucifix, which had great significance to me, on top of all the letters, and again took up the mantra: "I forgive you and bless you with love." But I still felt angry. I replaced the crucifix with a picture of a smiling Jesus, but that didn't work either. Finally I just disciplined myself to look at the photos and the letters, allowed myself to feel what I was feeling and to accept it, and then began saying the mantra again.

By staying with this new approach for a few hours, I was able to experience a peace settling over me along with the realization that "all is well." I continued to pronounce the blessing of forgiveness over and over during the course of the next day. Two days later, the Highway Patrol called and informed me that the accident report had been found. This was quickly followed by reimbursement for all of my "inconvenience" and payment in full for the purchase of a new car. On top of all that material reinforcement, I once again felt reconnected with my true self. This was my first conscious lesson in the positive, creative energy released through blessing.

Forgiveness must not be conceived as an act of condoning the poor behavior of another toward us, but rather as an act of release on our part in relation to the person we feel has harmed us. In that act of release, we place the individual into God's light and allow that light to dissolve the negative energy into which we once were plugged. Having unplugged psychically from past negative actions directed against us, we are now prepared to be filled with the positive energy of freedom and joy.

In the creation story of Genesis, God completed his work of creation by putting his stamp of approval on it with the words, "It is good." After creating man and woman, he looked upon all that had taken place and approved it by calling it "very good." In every situation and within each individual lies the inherent energy of goodness waiting to be released through blessings that declare, "It is good."

Simply to behold God in a person or situation is a blessing. When I pray for people, I generally do so in the form of a blessing.

Sometimes the blessing produces unusual manifestations of light and energy. This calls to mind the case of a woman named Dorothy, who along with her husband attended a healing prayer seminar I was conducting in Chicago at the beginning of 1995. Dorothy was not suffering from any particular physical ailment, but was someone who had a keen interest in spiritual matters and wanted to learn more about prayer. She later wrote to me to describe her experience:

"On Friday night, I felt 'power' in the room. I became very emotional and tears streamed quietly down my face. I felt as if huge hands had me sit up straight. There was a vibration across my pelvic region. I became aware of vibrations on the bottom of my feet and in the two small fingers on each hand, [as well as] the pelvic region, which [vibrations] moved up and through the stomach and then into my face. I became intensely hot yet did not perspire. My face blazed with color and there was tingling, pressure, and heat on my ears and the sides of my face along the cheekbone and temples. The backs of my eyes hurt like after the test for glaucoma.

"I became dizzy and went over to put my head on the open windowsill to get plenty of cold air. I stayed there a very long time. On the way home, as we were driving, the car filled with a fragrance I felt might be orange blossoms or oranges or peaches. It was pouring down rain and we could not explain the fragrance. I ate very little and went to bed at 8:30, totally exhausted. I slept without moving (rare for me) till 4:30 A.M. Rarely do I sleep more than five hours at one time. I fell asleep again until 6:30, ten hours all told—very rare for me. I did that only once before—after 36 hours on airplanes!

"[Following this experience] I spontaneously performed a healing for a headache, [and another] for a wrist pain due to a poor injection at the hospital. Both people said the pain was gone. I had never done healings before."

In this situation, I believe that Dorothy was being gifted with

Christ energy, which a few days later exhibited itself as a healing energy that brought relief to some of her acquaintances. The case of Dorothy is a classic example of someone with a heart that is open to the Christ energy receiving that energy and then turning around and applying it to serving others. She was anointed with Christedness and it manifested as healing energy both for her and through her. Dorothy, who had never previously experienced any desire to heal others, is now working as a spiritual healer in her own right, using prayer as a tool for healing with much success. She says that she has dedicated her life "to being a prayerful channel of God's healing love for people of all religious traditions and nonreligious backgrounds as well."

The prayer of blessing can be coupled with decree to become an even more powerful form of healing prayer. When God said, "Let there be light," he was in essence issuing a decree. The difference between blessing or decree and petition may seem slight, but it is all the difference in the world. When you decree a blessing by saying, "Let the Lord bless you now" or "The Lord's peace be on me," you are neither begging God to give you something nor telling Him to do something. Instead, you are calling down—on yourself or on whoever is the object of your blessing—the energy of God that is always present everywhere in the universe. The blessing given by God to Moses that I quoted earlier does not carry with it the burden of petition but rather the freedom of decree, and that is precisely why God gave that form to the priests of Israel. Decree is mentioned in the Book of Job (22:28): "Thou shalt also decree a thing, and it shall be established unto thee: and the light shall shine upon thy ways." The connection of the act of decreeing with light shining down is not, I think, accidental.

Some translations of scripture seem to enjoy decreasing the original energy released through decrees by replacing the decree or affirmation with a petition. As we have seen, this happened with the Lord's Prayer when it was translated from the Aramaic language of Jesus to Greek, Latin, Old English, and modern English. As the wording changed form, the energy inherent in the prayer diminished. Anyone disciplined in the area of conscious awareness can intuitively feel the different levels of energy that are released by petitioning as opposed to affirming something to be so. During petition, the energy level resembles the "flat line" on an ICU heart monitor—essentially dead. When decreeing a blessing, the energy profile increases to multiple impulses of a higher vibration. If you are "tuned in" to God's wavelength, you are able to feel the rise in energy on a physical level almost to the point where it is experienced as an accelerated heartbeat. So often in my work of spiritual healing through prayer therapy, people have expressed their experiences in just that way:

"When you blessed me, it felt like electricity was going through me."

"I felt electrified."

"I saw lots of lights around me."

"My body was tingling."

"I wasn't able to stand up."

"My body felt full of heat."

Blessing as prayer is a transmission of light-energy, which is why supernatural phenomena occur in the Bible when a blessing is spoken over a person or a group more than for other forms of prayer. In the Gospels, for example, Jesus spoke a blessing over the loaves and fishes and empowered the disciples to produce abundance. After Jesus had risen from the dead, he appeared to his disciples as they walked on the road to Emmaus. His disciples' faces were downcast as he talked to them, explaining the scriptures regarding Moses and the prophets. They later acknowledged that their hearts burned within them as Jesus talked, yet they didn't recognize Jesus until he blessed the bread with them. "Then their eyes were opened and they recognized him, and he vanished out of their sight" (Luke 24:18). I believe that at this time Jesus was fully illuminated and became so bright that the disciples literally could not see him.

As we discussed in an earlier chapter, by praying a blessing over the Israelites at the dedication of the Temple, Solomon caused fire to fall from heaven. Abram (whose name God later changed to Abraham) was in the process of becoming the father of a nation when Melchizedek, the priest-king of Salem, pronounced words of blessing over him. Afterward Abram's wife, Sarah, became pregnant at the age of ninety and Abram went on to be known as God's beloved.

Blessing is also a tool for healing, especially distant healing. Decreeing the accomplishment of God's favor brings positive results. When Catholic or Orthodox Christians bless, they often make the sign of the cross over what they are blessing to signify that the appearance of error or evil has been crossed out—making room for the appearance of good. This has been a ritual of mine for years when helping Christians who are in need of healing. Through the power released by the tremendous love involved in the historic event of the crucifixion, I decree the appearance of error crossed out, allowing for the sovereign will of God, which is divine health, to appear.

When Jesus healed the centurion's servant, the healing occurred at the very moment Jesus decreed him healed. There was no time or space between the declaration of the word and the healing, which is the way distant healing operates. Blessing as an affirmative decree is not conditioned by distance. We are all interconnected in the consciousness of God. When I think loving thoughts of God at the same time I think loving thoughts about an individual in need of God's healing love, we are spiritually connected and healing energy is released to all parties involved in an instant. "Bless a thing and it will bless you," goes an ancient proverb; "curse a thing and it will curse you."

I can attest to many remarkable results from such blessings and decrees. I must caution readers, however, not to assume that the practice of a certain religious ritual that brings miraculous results is proof of the correctness of that religion's beliefs and doctrine. I often practice a ritual simply because I am aware of the spiritual energy inherent in it and am comfortable with the ritual itself.

The forms of blessing and decree are related to the kind of authentic prayer I have been discussing in this book in a particular way that is embodied in the story of the Transfiguration. Authentic prayer is based on our receptivity to the light-energy of God. By opening ourselves to receive this energy, we become spiritually charged and open ourselves to spiritual, psychological, and physical healings of all kinds. But then what? If we look closely at the Transfiguration story, we see Jesus coming down from his mountaintop communion with the Father and immediately applying his regenerated powers in a healing of some magnitude. That is precisely what we are to do. We can begin by praying and calling down blessings on ourselves, but then we must move on to helping others to heal.

A word of caution is in order here. Be mindful that you can also decree the negative to come to pass in your life if you keep focusing on what you don't want or most fear. That decree also carries an authority to produce results. If you notice that your life is encased in negative energy, take note of what you are saying. Be aware, too, that what you decree does not always come from what you verbalize but sometimes from your constant thoughts. As you think, so shall you be, for better or worse.

In Mark 11:22–33, Jesus emphasizes the importance of the faith of God coupled with speaking with authority, implying that the speaking emerges naturally from our thought life. Before we speak, a thought is formed that springs forth from our belief system. Sensitive clairvoyants such as Annie Besant and C.W. Leadbeater have long claimed that they could actually *see* thought-forms as variously shaped and colored elements emerging from the aura of individual thinkers—their thoughts, in a sense, taking on a life of their own. When connected with God's love and faith, the energy generated by our thoughts creates good. When God spoke the words of creation in Genesis, He was filled with loving thoughts that were formed by His belief in good. Speaking the created words out of faith, the energy of the Holy Spirit created the universe. God knew He could create good. Made in God's likeness, we must come to the awareness that we, too, can create good. Indeed, we can cocreate good because the essence of God's Spirit dwells within us and is always available to us. But if we are careless in our thoughts, letting negative, uncharitable, or destructive fantasies take root in our psyches willy-nilly, we will also be responsible for the spiritual damage they may do.

The complete mystic, leaving everything to God's will, does not leave anything to chance, including his or her innermost thoughts. This does not mean, of course, that you may not experience all kinds of *feelings*—of anger, fear, lust, greed, even hatred. When they arise, watch them come and go, but don't invite them to stay. There is a big difference between feeling a surge of anger at someone who upsets you and dwelling in your rage so that it generates retributive impulses toward that person. If such feelings persist, take them into your daily prayer sessions and let the light of the Holy Spirit help to dissolve them.

The beauty of stories concerning Jesus' manifestation of prayer energy lies in the realization that we can live with the same conscious-

Jesus moved, and so produce the same results Jesus pro-
tter what our religious upbringing may be. Similar to
Jesus, we can become transformers or generators of the life force to a
world in pain. As we become more aware of our connection with God
through the various forms of blessing, we learn more about its importance to the healing of our lives and the lives of those around us.

EXERCISE FOR SELF-BLESSING

Blessing, like charity, begins at home—in this case, with self-
blessing. Once you have mastered that, you can begin to call down
blessings on others. So begin by sitting in your chair or meditation
place and taking three deep breaths. Read the blessing from the
Book of Numbers in either of the versions given earlier in this
chapter, substituting first-person pronouns for the second person
of the original. This might come out as follows:

> *The Lord bless me, the Lord keep me:*
> *The Lord make his face to shine upon me, and the Lord be*
> *gracious unto me:*
> *The Lord turn his face toward me and grant me peace and*
> *completeness in all areas of my life and on all levels of my*
> *being. Amen.*

When saying the blessing, pronounce it slowly and distinctly,
and say it out loud if circumstances permit. Recall that "Amen" in its
original form means "God is faithful." Have faith that God will
deliver this blessing to you.

Dan Millman, author of *The Way of the Peaceful Warrior* and other
books, suggests the use of what he calls "inner blessings"—silently
calling blessings down on the people with whom we interact

briefly, such as at the bank or office or grocery store. That's a fine idea, but if it seems overwhelming to try to remember to call down blessings on each interaction, you may find it more effective to announce your intention to do so during your morning or evening prayer session. If an especially upsetting encounter threatens to unbalance your equilibrium, of course, it may be helpful to stop, take a few deep breaths, and consciously bless the person with whom you're having a hard time. Besides helping prevent any spiritual damage, this technique may also keep you from escalating a bad situation into something you'll regret.

The Aramaic scholar Neil Douglas-Klotz offers his own expansion of the biblical blessing, based on a translation of a blessing from the Qumran community of the Dead Sea, which flourished between 100 B.C. and A.D. 100. He calls it "A Blessing of Lucid Fire and Secret Grace," and I find its language especially appropriate to our discussion of prayer and blessing and God as light-energy. You can apply this version to self-blessing by once again changing the pronouns appropriately, but you may also find it useful as is for announcing your intention to call down blessings on the people you will meet during the day's journey.

> *May the Being of the Universe*
> *breathe into you the light of blessing and ripeness,*
> *the fulfillment of health and balance;*
>
> *May it protect you from*
> *distractions brittle and bent*
> *with a sphere of lucid fire;*
>
> *May it enlighten*
> *the heart of your passion*
> *with the contemplation of living energy;*

May it uncover the
hidden strength within you,
insight gathered from the eternal now;

And may it show you its face
of secret grace and silent refuge
in a communion of deep peace.

TWELVE

TOWARD A DAILY MYSTICAL PRACTICE

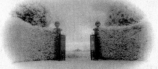

Ordinary people can and do become whole. They can and do live in ways that express their highest and most cherished values—values which also happen to be those most prized universally and collectively throughout human history. People who become whole are the ones who find completeness by consciously integrating inner and outer realities.

◆

MARSHA SINETAR, *ORDINARY PEOPLE AS MONKS AND MYSTICS*

H aving read through this book with some expectation of seeing a clear path laid out before you—a guideline to creating your own spiritual practice on a daily basis—you may be wondering exactly where to begin. I can relate to your dilemma because I've been in that situation myself, and for me, a rocking chair became the chief stimulus to remember to pray and bless.

I had been living the life of a parish priest and saying daily mass, but had pretty much given up saying the Daily Office, the cycle of prayers that all priests are supposed to recite throughout the day. The Office probably reaches back to the earliest days of the Desert Fathers and the Christian mystics of Egypt and Syria, who developed ways to pray continually, and it might seem like a pretty good model of daily mystical practice. I had begun, however, to find the prescribed prayers of the Office rather meaningless compared to the way I was learning to pray on my own. In the rectory, I used to pray occasionally in my bedroom, yet I had still not developed a regular meditative prayer life. There was a small den just off my bedroom that might have made a good prayer room, but that was where I also watched TV and it didn't seem very conducive to prayer.

I decided to make a commitment to pray for an hour each day, gathered all my prayer books and missals and rosaries and other prayer tools and spread them out around me, took a deep breath, closed my eyes, and started praying. I was enthusiastically committed to going the whole hour without stopping. After what seemed like a minor eternity, I opened my eyes with a great sense of gratitude in my heart for what I had just accomplished. Then I looked at my wristwatch and discovered that exactly seven minutes had gone by. I knew I was in deep trouble in my understanding of prayer.

That experience, however, led me to examine my frustration along with my unrealistic expectations. I was compelled to come to terms with my imperfect nature and to let it be okay that I wasn't yet a fully realized mystic! I knew that I liked having a prayer time apart from my priestly duties, but scaled back what I expected of myself. Over the weeks and months that followed, that first seven-minute period built to fifteen minutes, then twenty, then thirty minutes, an hour, and, after many months, sometimes two hours at a stretch. I didn't set out to sit that long, but I found myself enjoying the process so much that I often didn't notice the time. I certainly experienced days when I had trouble focusing, or when even half an hour seemed to drag by and I felt uninspired. But I also began to see results in my daily life in the form of generally increasing patience and a sense of equanimity.

After I had overcome my resistance to sitting for more than a few minutes, however, I began to realize that one long session in the morning, or even two sessions bookending my days, was not enough, because they still left a long block of time during which I could forget about God altogether. Around the time I came to this realization, I happened to put an old rocking chair in the corner of my bedroom that I was using for prayer. As soon as I did, I noticed a subtle yet profound change in my day. Now whenever I went past the room, I would see the rocker and stop to sit in it for a minute or two. It looked so inviting, why not take a short break there in the middle of the day? That small change helped my unconscious develop an awareness of God that spread throughout the entire day. It got to where just looking at the rocking chair was enough to remind me of God's presence. The gaps in my awareness gradually began to disappear.

I tell this story not only to show that my own development of a daily practice was slow and stepwise, but also that you can never know what will act as the catalyst to getting serious about praying. Just as some prayers or exercises may work well for certain people but not for others, the same is true for prayer routines and the environment in which you pray. Most meditation teachers recommend designating a separate room for sitting each day, but that may not always be possible, especially if you live in a small apartment or have children around. Still, most people can find at least a corner of their bedroom that will do in a pinch. All you really need is a cushion or a chair to sit on, a tape player if you want to listen to music or meditation tapes, and perhaps a few sacred images.

Don't be afraid to mix images from different religious traditions if this appeals to you. The shrine room has long been a fixture of Asian households, where figures from Taoist, Confucianist, and Buddhist iconography traditionally share the same space. If you prefer images of the Divine Feminine, there are plenty to choose from, starting with Mother Mary, Saint Teresa, or Saint Clare, Kuan Yin from the Chinese tradition, any of the forms of Tibetan Tara, copies of ancient Mother Goddess figurines, or images of the feminine energy principle known as Shakti from India in the form of the goddesses Kali, Durga, Uma, and many more. There's no reason why you can't also include photos of departed parents or loved ones if they inspire you.

Images of living teachers are appropriate as well if you feel a connection to them. Especially in the beginning, though, you may want to focus mainly on one tradition in terms of the practice itself. Swami Muktananda used to liken the search for a spiritual path to looking for water in your backyard. Some seekers, he said, run around digging one hole after another, each a few feet deep, and then feel frustrated when they don't find water. You have to choose one spot and dig down as deep as you can go, Muktananda said, if you want to make a real well and reach the groundwater that's down there. Any genuine spiritual master will probably agree that it makes little difference which path you choose to follow; all can lead you to a realization of God in your life. The important thing is to choose one and stick with it long enough to achieve the kind of genuine depth that can result in opening your heart. Trying a Zen approach one month, Kabbalah the next, then a few months of Vedanta followed by Goddess worship probably won't help you feel fulfilled. It's all too easy to get stuck in what the Tibetan Buddhist teacher and author Chogyam Trungpa Rinpoche aptly dubbed "spiritual materialism," which he likened to collecting beautiful antiques. "We could be specializing in oriental antiques," Trungpa wrote, "or medieval Christian antiques or antiques from some other civilization or time, but we are, nonetheless, running a shop."

Having said that, I want to reiterate how strongly I believe that inspiration and guidance can come to us from a multitude of spiritual teachers of all the world's wisdom traditions. One of the richest sources of their wisdom, of course, is their writings. Good spiritual books from any tradition can be a great help in leading you into a meditation or prayer session. It doesn't much matter if the book is by a Vietnamese Buddhist monk or an American Jewish popularizer, because reading just a page or two or as little as a few lines can give you a new perspective when you're feeling stuck.

It's hard for me to wander through the aisles of any good spiritual bookstore, or the religion and spirituality section of a large bookstore, without feeling drawn to one or more books. And maybe "drawn" is the key word here. When it comes to crafting a daily practice for yourself, one of the most helpful guides is your own intuition. I suggest that you allow your intuition to be guided by God's Spirit to the books, tapes, and teachers that are right for you at this point in your walk. You can do this by inviting the Holy Spirit to guide you as a shepherd guides his flock. Various coincidences (not accidents) will seem to pop up in your life, leading you to where God wants you to go.

I recall a difficult period in my life when everything came crashing down and a sense of depression completely overwhelmed me. Yet in the midst of all that confusion, I heard a voice within me tell me to take a walk through the bookstore located near my residence. I didn't want to—I would much rather have stayed home and wallowed in self-pity—but I obeyed. As I walked the aisles of the bookstore, a book caught my eye. Its title shouted out to me, "Help, my life hurts!" After purchasing the book and digesting its contents, I began to feel much better and the depression began to leave. Coincidence? Accident? This was the guidance of God, assisting my return to equanimity. Today I can't even recall the exact title of the book or its author; a while back I gave it to a friend who was experiencing similar turmoil in his life, and I've since lost track of it. But it was there when I needed help, and my inner voice led me to it. Be aware of that small voice of guidance, because it comes from a big God.

I didn't just read or study that book, by the way. I picked out phrases that meant something to me and pondered them meditatively until they became part of me. In doing so, I came to feel God and know His love for me. I was filled with gratitude for being led to that book. So when an impulse leads you to a book under such circumstances, or to a picture or a tape, I recommend that you take it into your place of prayer and incorporate it in your daily practice for as long as it feels right to do so. I'm not suggesting that you substitute reading for prayer, simply that you use whatever comes to hand. You may find it more helpful to chant (whether in English, Latin, Sanskrit, Japanese, or Yoruba matters only to you), or to listen silently to music of your choice. Some people may be more comfortable mixing these approaches, letting themselves be guided each day whether to read, chant, pray, or meditate silently. Others will prefer developing a fixed routine over time and then sticking to that.

Whatever choices you make, however, expect a certain amount of resistance. You may wonder why, if daily practice is such a good idea, you find it so difficult at times to stick to it. That's the voice of your ego, the separative aspect of your nature that has evolved over millions of years with only one goal in mind: survival. Although we can recognize and appreciate the value of a strong survival instinct, especially in that moment when we find ourselves standing in the path of an oncoming Mack truck, we also have to understand its limitations. We have to be clear that the ego ultimately must take a backseat to spiritual advancement. "He who would save his life must lose it" was not just a clever aphorism tossed off by a desert teacher from Galilee. Jesus meant precisely that we have to throw away certain aspects of our survival instinct—our ego—if we are ever going to enter the kingdom.

In time we may be able to view the ego as a friendly adversary, rather than attacking our survival instincts the way many ascetics have done. That path, as the Buddha discovered 2,500 years ago, rarely works. The Middle Way he developed, between aversion to the senses and enslavement to them—in Christian parlance, being in the world but not of the world—works much better for most of us. Still, your ego will see no benefit in a continued spiritual practice the very goal of which is to dissolve the ego in the light of the Holy Spirit. Despite the fact that regular meditation may, as a byproduct, lower your blood pressure, relieve stress, and perhaps help you live a little longer, your ego won't really care since it will be afraid that it won't be around to enjoy the fruits of all that. The ego is a little like HAL the Computer in the movie *2001: A Space Odyssey*. Once it senses that the person in charge has discovered that its guidance system is flawed and its days are numbered, it will fight with every tool at its disposal to prevent its own dismemberment—even if that means killing off its chances for joy in the process.

So humor your ego but don't let it call the shots. If you start feeling too much resistance, cut back a little on your daily time, but don't give up on it altogether. It's better to pray for ten minutes a day every day of the week than to sit for two or three hours every once in a while. That's where the institutional religions went off the tracks in the first place. Being a mystic means nothing if not taking a holistic approach to spirituality. Even though, in an absolute sense, time does not exist, here on earth we have very limited time to effect major changes in ourselves and those around us. Begrudging a few minutes a day to keep spiritually focused is just another form of poverty mentality, the equivalent of saying, I don't have enough time to do my work, enjoy my life, and still keep my mind and heart centered on God.

In a sense, of course, you have nothing *but* time. Don't fall into the trap of thinking of your practice as something that happens for thirty minutes or an hour every morning or evening. Genuine mysticism means always finding ways to bring your attention back to God, always discerning the workings of the Holy Spirit in the world as you pass through it. It is this continuity, this constant maintenance of awareness, that should really be your goal. I've suggested a number of ways throughout this book to bring your remembrance back to the Divine in the course of the day. It doesn't much matter whether you use prayer beads, notes, a wristwatch, observations of nature, or a string tied around your finger, as long as it works for you. That's only a beginning mechanism in any event, some way to start training your consciousness to work for you instead of against you. Once you've learned to begin exercising your will to pray without ceasing, your imagination will open up new roadways for you. Try as your ego may, it will finally be no match for the divine energy that will flow into you as a result.

ADDITIONAL PRAYERS FOR USE AS YOU SEE FIT

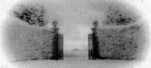

And in praying do not heap up empty phrases as the Gentiles do; for they think that they will be heard for their many words. Do not be like them, for your Father knows what you need before you ask him.

◆

MATTHEW 6:7–8

The world is full of wonderful prayers that are rarely spoken outside of religious orders or institutions of various sorts. Although I generally prefer prayer that comes spontaneously from the heart or that contains no words at all, I often find these other prayers can have the power to inspire the soul and warm the heart. Especially when you may be feeling at a loss for words or may be having difficulty starting your daily practice, reading one of these prayers in a deliberate and heartfelt manner and pondering their words may help you get going. They come from a wide variety of traditions and sources, so feel free to substitute names for the Absolute with those which you may feel more at home, or to change the gender or number of the personal pronouns in them.

Cardinal Newman's Prayer

Cardinal John Henry Newman (1801–1890), who came from a British family with Evangelical sympathies, became active in the Anglican Church before becoming a Roman Catholic in 1845. His prayer is now said daily by Mother Teresa's Missionaries of Charity. What appeals to me most about it is the clear evocation of the Christ as light-energy that shines through us as we make ourselves yielded vessels for God's work.

> Dear Jesus, help us (me) to spread your fragrance everywhere we (I) go. Flood our souls with your spirit and life. Penetrate and possess our whole being so utterly that our lives may only be a radiance of yours. Shine

through us, and be so in us, that every soul we come in contact with may feel your presence in our soul. Let them look up and see no longer us but only Jesus! Stay with us, and then we shall begin to shine as you shine; so to share as to be a light to others; the light, O Jesus, will be all from you, none of it will be ours; it will be you, shining on others through us. Let us preach you without preaching, not by words but by our example, by the catching force, the sympathetic influence of what we do, the evident fullness of the love our hearts bear to you.

Expanded Prayer for Protection

The Unity School of Christianity, or Unity, is not a church but a nonsectarian educational organization whose founders were influenced by Christian Science, Quakerism, Theosophy, and Hinduism. James Dillet Freeman (b. 1912), a prominent member of Unity for many years, composed the original five-line Prayer for Protection in 1941 (astronaut Edwin "Buzz" Aldrin carried it with him to the moon). However, I prefer this expanded version, the author of which is to the best of my knowledge unknown.

The Light of God surrounds me.
The Love of God enfolds me.
The Power of God protects me.
The Presence of God watches over me.

The Mind of God guides me.
The Life of God flows through me.
The Laws of God direct me.
The Power of God abides within me.
The Joy of God uplifts me.
The Strength of God renews me.
The Beauty of God inspires me.
Wherever I am, God is!
And all is well.

Prayer of Saint Francis

To my mind, the true test of all great mystics and spiritual teachers is whether the essence of their life and teachings is compassion. Saint Francis of Assisi (c. 1181–1226), the son of a wealthy Italian silk merchant, lived an extravagant, carefree life until his visions of Christ led him to devote himself to the care of the poor and sick—causing his father to disinherit him. Francis's compassion and his sense of being a conduit of God's healing grace make him a role model of authentic prayer. He wrote many prayers, but this is his best known, and justly so.

Lord, make me an instrument of your peace.
Where there is hatred, let me sow love;
where there is injury, pardon;
where there is doubt, faith;
where there is despair, hope;
where there is darkness, light;
and where there is sadness, joy.

O, Lord, grant that I may not so much
seek to be consoled as to console;
to be understood as to understand;
to be loved as to love;
for it is in giving that we receive;
it is in pardoning that we are pardoned, and it is in
dying that we are
born to eternal life.

Evening Prayer

The Sikh religion came into being in the sixteenth century with the idea of dissolving the differences between Hindus and Muslims and among India's castes. Sikhism incorporates elements of Eastern and Western theology; it is essentially monotheistic yet its goal is union with God, who is said to dwell in each human being. Sikhs accept the principles of karma and reincarnation, yet insist on the equality of all castes and of women. This excerpt from the Evening Prayer comes from their sacred text known as the Adi Granth, translated by Khushwant Singh.

On hearing of the Lord,
All men speak of His greatness;
Only he that hath seen Him
Can know how great is He.
Who can conceive of His worth
Or who can describe Him?
Those who seek to describe Thee
Are lost in Thy depths.

Releasing Healing Energy Through Sacred Verses

The word "inspire" literally means "to breathe in," and all the sacred scriptures of the world contain inspired writings that have been breathed into the writers by the Holy Spirit. When you read them, you can release that sacred energy into your own heart and soul, which is just another way of saying that the verses themselves carry a sacred vibration. Even if you don't read them in the original language, that energy is available to you. I recommend that you choose one of the following verses for each prayer session and let it resonate within you.

Start, for example, with this verse: "Pleasant words are like a honeycomb sweetness to the soul (inner being), and health (healing) to the bones" (Prov. 16:24, my parentheses). Put on a tape of soft harp music or chanting, and if you have an aromatherapy disperser, use a sweet smell that appeals to you and puts you in a meditative state, such as honeysuckle or orange blossom. (You can also use incense if the smoke doesn't bother you.) Then slowly recite the words out loud or silently. After reading the whole proverb gently, offer some words of your own in a whisper: love, peace, bliss. Choose words that have for you the sweetness of a honeycomb.

This process is what I mean by being holistic. Use the senses God has given you to bring in health and healing—sight, sound, smell—along with mental concentration and the intention to open your heart.

Here are some other scriptural selections from the Jewish-Christian tradition to begin with.

> God, who raised Jesus from the dead, will also give life
> to your mortal bodies through His Spirit who dwells
> within (Rom. 8:11).

God says, "I know the thoughts and plans I have for you. Plans to bring you hope, peace and give you a future" (Jer. 29:11).

The leper came to Jesus and said, "Lord if you want to, you can heal me" and Jesus said, "I want to—be healed" (Matt. 8:2,3).

Praise the Lord with affection and do not forget God's blessings and benefits, for He forgives all your iniquities and heals all your diseases (Ps. 103:1–3).

He sent His word and healed them and delivered them from what was destroying them (Ps. 107:20).

Beloved, I desire above all else that you may prosper and be in health even as your soul prospers (3 John 2).

This is a holistic decree if I've ever seen one. If you are saying this for someone else, insert their name(s) at the beginning. If you want to use it for yourself, change the pronouns to first person. If possible, have someone who knows that God is a good God and acts on that in a positive manner lay hands on you and anoint you with oil. Let the person pray over you while decreeing the above statement.

At the end of the ritual, you may decree, "This affliction will not rise up again" (Nah. 1:9).

From the Hindu tradition of India:

May our ears hear the good, may our eyes see the good. May we serve Him with the full strength of our body. May we all our life carry out His will. May peace and peace and peace be everywhere.

MUNDAKA UPAMISHAD
(TRANSLATED BY W. B. YEATS
AND SHREE PUROHIT SWAMI)

God ended his work and rested, and he made a bond of love between his soul and the soul of all things. And the One became one with the One.

SVATASVATARA UPANISHAD
(TRANSLATED BY JUAN MASCARÓ)

The light of the Atman, the Spirit, is invisible, concealed in all beings. It is seen by the seers of the subtle, when their vision is keen and clear. . . .

Awake, arise! Strive for the Highest, and be in the Light! Sages say the path is narrow and difficult to tread, narrow as the edge of a razor.

KATHA UPANISHAD
(TRANSLATED BY JUAN MASCARÓ)

In the Bhagavad Gita, the Lord speaks to Arjuna: "Those intent on Me who dedicate all their rituals and work to Me, who meditate on Me, who revere Me, them I lift up. Keep your mind centered on Me."

From the Buddhist tradition:

Ah, happily do we live in good health among the ailing; amidst the ailing we dwell in good health.

From the Taoist tradition of China:

> *I have just three things to teach:*
> *simplicity, patience, compassion.*
> *These three are your greatest treasures.*
> *Simple in actions and in thoughts,*
> *you return to the source of being.*
> *Patient with both friends and enemies,*
> *you accord with the way things are.*
> *Compassionate toward yourself,*
> *you reconcile all beings in the world.*

TAO TE CHING 67
(TRANSLATED BY STEPHEN MITCHELL)

From the Islamic tradition:

> God (Allah) is the light of the heavens and the earth. His light may be compared to a niche that enshrines a lamp, the lamp within a crystal of star-like brilliance. It is lit from a blessed olive tree neither eastern nor western. Its very oil would almost shine forth, though no fire touched it. Light upon light; God guides to His light whom He will.

QURAN 24:35
(TRANSLATED BY N.J. DAWOOD)

The religion of love is separate from all religions.
The loves of God have no religion but God alone.
Light up a fire of love in your soul, burn all thought and
   expression away.

JELALUDDIN RUMI (1207–1273),
"THE SHEPHERD'S PRAYER"

From the Gnostic tradition of the Nag Hammadi Library:

> It is not possible for anyone to see anything of the things that actually exist unless he becomes like them.
> This is quite in keeping with the truth. You saw the Spirit, you became Spirit. You saw Christ, you became Christ. You saw the Father, you shall become the Father.
>
> GOSPEL OF PHILIP

Praying the Names of God

> *Contemplate solely the Name of God—*
> *Fruitless are all other rituals.*
>
> ADI GRANTH (SIKHISM)

In all the ancient religions, the most important form of prayer was the prayer of the names of God. When you learn to say the name of God as a prayer, especially in conjunction with the use of any picture that for you contains the energy of God's personality, you can begin to feel the power of that prayer throughout your being. Hindus and Muslims use prayer beads to count as they repeat the names of God. I use a Catholic rosary, not often to pray the traditional form but to pronounce names of God. In the following exercise, we are going to use various names of God, and if I happen to miss yours, please understand that I haven't done so on purpose.

Take a deep breath and relax your body. Take another deep breath and relax your thoughts. Then take one more deep breath to enter into your spiritual kingdom, your true essence. Close your eyes and symbolically block out everything else with the commitment that what you want more than anything is God.

O pure Being, Source of all life, my Mother, Father, Creator of the Cosmos, you who are perfect Goodness and absolute Love, we open our whole being to you for the inrushing of your divine Spirit, your divine energy, your divine presence. Lord, taking our hint from the past, we begin to invoke your presence by chanting and concentrating on your many beautiful names.

In all the ancient spiritual languages, the sound of "ah" was common to the names of God, either at the beginning of the name, as the name itself, or at the end. And so now take a deep breath and let the sound "ahhhh" come out of your mouth as you exhale. Take a deep breath and stretch it out this time: ahhhhhhhhhhhhhhhhhh.

Now let's raise it a level. Take a deep breath and exhale at a slightly higher pitch: ahhhhhhhh. Take another deep breath and let it out again: ahhhhhhhh. Now just breathe normally, take your little finger and ring finger, press them against your thumb, and place your hand on your heart. Take a deep breath and exhale.

Now take a deep breath and this time exhale the name of God in Aramaic, *Alaha,* stretching it out to sound like ahhhh-laaaa-haaaa. Repeat the name two more times. Then take a deep breath, and this time say the name in Arabic, *Allah:* Ahhhh-lahhhh. Again and with each new name, repeat it twice more. Then take a deep breath, and this time say the name in Hebrew, *Yahweh:* Yahhhh-wehhhh.

There were many names for the Goddess, the Source of all life, in the ancient religions of the Middle East, including Astarte, Ishtar, and Inanna. Choosing one, take a deep breath and exhale: In-ahhhh-nahhhh. Or chant: Ahhhh-stahhhhr-tehhhh.

Now take a deep breath and say the name of Jesus in Aramaic: *Yeshua:* Yehhhh-shuuuu-wahhhh. Take another deep breath and say one of the many names of God in Sanskrit, *Krishna:*

Krishhhh-nahhhh. Be aware of the vibrations going on in your body, especially in the area where your fingers and thumb are over your heart.

Technically, Buddha ("Awakened One") is not a name of God, yet the Buddha in several different manifestations is revered by Buddhists the world over with very much the same reverence others show to God. In Sanskrit, the first syllable of his name rhymes with "good," and the second syllable begins with *h:* Buuuud-haaaa.

HEALING
PRAYERS

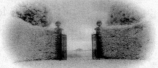

There has come to you an exhortation from your Lord, a balm for that which is in the breasts, a guidance and mercy for believers.

◆

QURAN 10:57

In the messianic future, the Holy One will heal the injury [of Adam's sin]. He will heal the wound of the world.

◆

TALMUD, GENESIS RABBAH 10:4

I composed the following prayers in response to specific calls from people asking for healing. Once again, you can use these as you feel the need, but I also encourage you to use them in another sense as models for your own prayers. As the Buddha said of his teachings, they are a raft to help ferry you to the far shore. Use the raft to cross over the river, but don't carry it on your back for the rest of your life.

Everlasting and eternal God, each time I come to you for this time of intimacy, this time of communion, this time of prayer, it is the start of a new spiritual day. With the warmth of your everlasting light, love, and mercy filling me, I feel awakened in my consciousness to your very presence, which removes the darkness of doubt and fear that encompass me in my time of need. Now I sense in the bright light of your Holy Spirit your majesty, presence, and healing power. My faith in you, Lord, and in your love is renewed as I become one with you. I open my heart, my soul, my spirit, my body, my whole being, and my life to your healing presence. I am being renewed now in this presence. Amen. So be it. God is faithful.

Lord God, you are the healer of my soul, my spirit, and my body. You truly desire the best for all your children. You desire to give me a future and a hope by healing every manner of sickness and disease, by strengthening, curing, comforting, and consoling me. Lord, it is your perfect will, your greatest desire to see your children healthy and whole, filled with the joy of your Spirit. I thank you, my Divine Parent.

Lord, you are the enemy of death and disease and in and through your Spirit disease, death, illness, broken relationships, and all other difficulties and problems are overcome and conquered. God, you lay your healing hands upon me now that I may feel the waves of energy saturating me, surrounding me, and bathing everything with light. You are faithful, Lord. Thank you.

O wonderful Lord, God, who sent forth His Spirit, His very Breath of life, I feel you now. As I sense your presence, I sense my fragmentation disappearing. I am becoming aware of wholeness returning to me. Within me joy wells up and signals that your presence is at work healing and restoring. Indeed, I, who have felt like the desert—bleached, parched, and wearied—am now coming alive. I feel the life of the Spirit within me bursting forth. You are a wonderful God and to you I am so grateful. Thank you for your healing presence.

In the light of your wonderful, healing Spirit, I sense your love, your mercy, and your compassion. Living in this light, I sense your special presence. This light and this presence exude tremendous power, the power of the Spirit to heal.

This light casts no shadow. It is perfectly pure with no darkness in it. As your light enters into my body, it removes all darkness, for wherever the light is, darkness cannot remain. Disease is darkness. Light is the love and mercy that heals. The very light of God, the very healing power and presence of God now cover the darkness and it disappears. It no longer exists. For this I am grateful, Lord. You are blessing your child now with healing of the body, the soul, and the Spirit. So be it.

Wonderful Lord God, Father, Mother, eternal mystery, divine healing presence, I believe in your boundless, unchanging love. My Divine Parent, I intend to forget the past and I no longer desire to focus on the future with fear and anxiety. I want to live this present moment in peace, in your presence, knowing that you are for me and not against me. I rest in the awareness of your love and mercy. United with your presence and your power, I am filled with gratitude. Thank you for the good you are bringing into my life this very moment. I am confident of this one thing, that you, who have begun this good work in me, are bringing it to completion. So be it. God is faithful.

Dearest Father, Mother, God, I feel the approaching presence of your Holy Spirit like electrical vibrations moving up and down my body, in and out and around my body. I approach you in loving embrace and in that embrace, I sense your merciful presence pouring through me. I'm entering an envelope of protection by entering your light of healing. I feel it moving, not only toward me but throughout my whole being. I sense that light now, replacing the darkness that is within me, going to the place that is most in need of your divine energy, resurrecting into new health that which is sick in me. O precious Spirit of the living God, Breath of life that raised Jesus from the dead, you are raising me up into a new life, a new awareness of your love and mercy that heals. I accept it! I receive it right now, for you love me unconditionally and for this I am grateful.

I reach out now, Lord, to the healing waters of your Spirit, allowing those healing waters to overflow and overwhelm me as I rest in your presence, as I sense your peace. For this I am grateful, so be it. I truly feel that all is well in my world, for you are a God who is not displeased with me. You are a God who desires to pour out your love on me, the love that heals like an anointing oil. I intend to receive all that you desire to give me. So be it. Amen. Thank you for being there for me.

Dear God, I come to you that I may drink of the living waters that flow from your fountain of life. These waters have the power to cleanse, to purify, to refresh, to revive, to make me whole. I am now being filled to overflowing with the waters of your spiritual healing power. The power that flows, the water that flows from your Spirit, your Breath of life, Lord God, I drink of it now and it is making me whole. I feel such a joy to be able to participate in this healing, Lord, that you are working in me now. For this I am grateful and I thank you.

O God of might, O God of heavenly power, Creator of the whole universe, one word from you can free us from every weakness and disease. I know, Father, because of your love you hear my prayer during my time of communion with you this day. Now through the flow of your Holy Spirit, you free me from my sickness, you restore me to health, and you give me the vigor and strength to live life to the fullest. Amen. So be it.

Infinite Creator of the Cosmos, Mother of all life, my greatest intention is to feel the vital breath of your healing Spirit upon me, driving from me all the fog that has obscured my vision in the past. My greatest hope, my greatest desire, my greatest intention right now is to come fully into your healing presence with an awareness of all your magnificence saturating me, surrounding me, and bathing everything with light. Thank you, God, for being so faithful and sure to your promises.

The following Faith Declarations are based on quotations from the Old and New Testaments and may be said after any of the Healing Prayers.

I am complete in Him who is the head of all principality and power (Col. 2:10).

I am far from oppression, and fear does not come near me (Isa. 54:14).

I am holy and without blame before Him in love (1 Pet. 1:16; Eph. 1:4).

I have the mind of the Christ (Phil. 2:5; 1 Cor. 2:16).

I have the peace of God that passes understanding (Phil. 4:7).

I have the Greater One living in me; greater is He who is in me than he who is in the world (1 John 4:4).

I have received the Spirit of wisdom and revelation in the knowledge of Jesus and the eyes of my understanding are enlightened (Eph. 1:17–18).

I have received the power of the Holy Spirit; to lay hands on the sick and see them recover, to cast out demons, to speak with new tongues; I have power over all the power of the enemy and nothing shall by any means harm me (Mark 16:17, 18; Luke 10:17, 19).

I have no lack for my God supplies all of my needs according to His riches (Phil. 4:19).

I show forth the praises of God, who has called me out of darkness into His marvelous light (1 Pet. 2:9).

I am God's child, for I am born again of the incorruptible seed of the Word of God, which lives and abides forever (1 Pet. 1:23).

I am part of a chosen generation, a royal priesthood, a holy nation, a purchased people (1 Pet. 2:9).

I am the temple of the Holy Spirit; I am not my own (1 Cor. 6:19).

I am the light of the world (Matt. 5:14).

I am His elect, full of mercy, kindness, humility and patience (Col. 3:12; Rom. 8:33).

I am delivered from the power of darkness and translated into God's kingdom (Col. 1:13).

I am firmly rooted, built up, established in my faith and overflowing with gratitude (Col. 2:7).

I am greatly loved by God (Col. 3:12; Rom. 1:7; 1 Thess. 1:4; Eph. 2:4).

SELECTED BIBLIOGRAPHY

◆

A Course in Miracles. Glen Ellen, Calif.: Foundation for Inner Peace, 1992.

The Amplified Bible. Grand Rapids, Mich.: Zondervan Publishing House, 1965.

Besant, Annie, and C.W. Leadbeater. *Thought-Forms.* Wheaton, Illinois: Theosophical Publishing House, 1969. (Originally published 1901.)

Douglas-Klotz, Neil. *Desert Wisdom: Sacred Middle-Eastern Writings from the Goddess Through the Sufis.* San Francisco: Harper San Francisco, 1995.

———. *Prayers of the Cosmos: Meditations on the Aramaic Words of Jesus.* San Francisco: Harper San Francisco, 1990.

Dyer, Wayne W. *Real Magic: Creating Miracles in Everyday Life.* New York: HarperCollins, 1992.

Epstein, Daniel Mark. *Sister Aimee: The Life of Aimee Semple McPherson.* New York: Harcourt Brace Jovanovich, 1993.

Errico, Rocco A. *The Ancient Aramaic Prayers of Jesus: "The Lord's Prayer."* Los Angeles: Science of Mind Publications, 1978.

Fox, Matthew. *Illuminations of Hildegard of Bingen.* Santa Fe: Bear & Co., 1985.

Griffiths, Bede. *Universal Wisdom: A Journey Through the Sacred Wisdom of the World.* San Francisco: Harper San Francisco, 1994.

Kuhlman, Kathryn. *God Can Do It Again.* N.J.: Bridge Publishing, 1993.

John G. Lake: His Life, His Sermons, His Boldness of Faith. Fort Worth, Tex.: Kenneth Copeland Publications, 1994.

Leadbeater, C.W. *The Science of the Sacraments.* Adyar, India: Theosophical Publishing House, 1975.

Liardon, Roberts. *God's Generals: Why They Succeeded and Why Some Failed.* Tulsa, Okla.: Albury Publishing, 1996.

Muktananda, Swami. *Play of Consciousness.* South Fallsburg, N.Y.: SYDA Foundation, 1978.

Occhiogrosso, Peter. *The Joy of Sects: A Spirited Guide to the World's Religious Traditions.* New York: Image Books,1996.

Parfitt, Will. *The New Living Qabalah: A Practical and Experiential Guide to Understanding the Tree of Life.* Rockport, Mass.: Element Books, 1991.

Pennington, Basil, O.C.S.O. *Centering Prayer: Renewing an Ancient Christian Prayer Form.* New York: Image Books, 1982.

Stratton, Elizabeth. *Touching Spirit: A Journey of Healing and Personal Resurrection.* New York: Simon & Schuster, 1996.

Strehlow, Widghard, Ph.D., and Gottfried Hertzka, M.D. *Hildegard of Bingen's Medicine.* Santa Fe: Bear & Co., 1988.

Warner, Wayne E. *Kathryn Kuhlman: The Woman Behind the Miracles.* Ann Arbor, Mich.: Servant Publications, 1993.

Wilson, Andrew, ed. *World Scripture: A Comparative Anthology of Sacred Texts.* New York: Paragon House, 1995.

Worrall, Ambrose A., and Olga N. Worrall. *The Gift of Healing: A Personal Story of Spiritual Therapy.* Columbus, Ohio: Ariel Press, 1985.

Yogananda, Paramahansa. *Autobiography of a Yogi.* Los Angeles: Self-Realization Fellowship, 1974. (Originally published 1946.)

Suggested Inspirational Reading

Bernardin, Joseph Cardinal. *The Gift of Peace: Personal Reflections.* Chicago: Loyola Press, 1997.

Broughton, Rosemary. *Praying with Teresa of Ávila.* Winona, Minn.: St. Mary's Press, 1990.

Cataneo, Pascal. *Padre Pio Gleanings.* Translated by Maureen McCollum and Gabriel Dextraze. Sherbrooke, Quebec, Canada: Editions Paulines, 1991.

Davis, Avram. *The Way of Flame: A Guide to the Forgotten Mystical Tradition of Jewish Meditation.* San Francisco: Harper San Francisco, 1996.

Durka, Gloria. *Praying with Hildegard of Bingen.* Winona, Minn.: St. Mary's Press, 1991.

Fox, Matthew. *Meditations with Meister Eckhart.* Santa Fe: Bear & Co., 1983.

Keating, Thomas. *Intimacy with God.* New York: Crossroads, 1995.

Mother Teresa: A Simple Path. Compiled by Lucinda Vardey. New York: Ballantine Books, 1995.

Nisargadatta Maharaj, Sri. *I Am That.* Translated by Maurice Frydman. Durham, N.C.: The Acorn Press, 1973.

O'Brien, Justin. *A Meeting of Mystic Paths: Christianity and Yoga.* St. Paul, Minn.: Yes International Publishers, 1996.

Sondweiss, Samuel, M.D. *Sai Baba the Holy Man . . . and the Psychiatrist.* San Diego: Birth Day Publishing, 1975.

Sanford, Agnes. *Behold Your God.* St. Paul, Minn.: Macalester Park Publishing, 1958.

————. *The Healing Light.* St. Paul, Minn.: Macalester Park Publishing, 1947.

Simsic, Wayne. *Praying with Thomas Merton.* Winona, Minn.: St. Mary's Press, 1994.

————. *Praying with John of the Cross.* Winona, Minn.: St. Mary's Press, 1993.

Sparrow, Scott. *Blessed Among Women: Encounters with Mary and Her Message.* New York: Harmony Books, 1997.

Worrall, Ambrose A., and Olga N. Worrall. *The Gift of Healing.* Columbus, Ohio: Ariel Press, 1985. (Originally published 1965.)

Yogananda, Paramahansa. *Divine Romance.* Los Angeles: Self-Realization Fellowship, 1986.

For more information on Ron Roth's spiritual healing retreats, Holistic Spirituality intensive workshops, and prayer seminars, you may write to him at Route 1, East Lynnewood, Peru, IL 61354, or fax him at (815) 224-3395. The following sets of audiotapes and videocassettes are also available:

Transformed by Love: The Healing Power of Authentic Self-Love

The Power of Prayer

Healing Prayers to Release the Power of God

Forgiveness Therapy: A Christ-Centered Approach

Prayer and the Rituals of Prayer as Energy Medicine

Holy Spirit: The Boundless Energy of God

Praying with Power for Healing, Guidance, Abundance, and Relationships (videocassettes)

Spiritual Healing: Merging Mysticism and Meditation with Medicine (videocassettes)

Ron is interested in hearing from readers who experience healing—whether physical, psychological, or spiritual—as a result of performing any of the prayer and meditation exercises or sacramental rituals described in this book, or from attending any of his healing services or workshops. You may write or fax him at the address or fax number given above.

INDEX

◆